Contents

Editorial

This collection of articles considers the issue of health from a gender perspective. What are the differences between women's and men's experiences of health, sickness, and health care, and how does our gender identity – and the roles which accompany this – affect our physical and mental wellbeing? Health, envisaged as total mental and physical wellbeing rather than a mere absence of illness, has been a major focus for the international women's movement from the 1970s onwards: 'It is a common recognition both of their need for control over their own bodies, and of the social origins of many of their health problems, that has led many women into political action. Physical and mental health are universal and basic needs.' (Doyal 1995, 7) Added to this there is growing interest in men's gendered health needs and interests – in particular concerning their mental health – among researchers in the fields of both health and masculinities.

Currently, although there have been improvements in various health indicators in many countries, developing countries are facing a health crisis. Many people in developing countries have never had access to formal medical services, while others have lost their access because of reductions in government spending as the result of structural adjustment packages, international debt repayments, and the deprioritising of health against other sectors. Although there

have been improvements in various health indicators in many countries, 11 million people die each year from infectious diseases – three million of them from AIDS (Oxfam 2000, 2). Drugs to address tropical diseases are not prioritised by the research and development depart-ments of drug companies, and diseases that *can* be treated by drugs often go uncontrolled because of the high and rising cost of drugs patented by western suppliers. International rules governing patents, laid down in TRIPS (the WTO agreement on Trade-Related Aspects of Intellectual Property Rights), provide legal frameworks binding countries to respect patent agreements, making it impossible to afford or manufacture vital medicines. New diseases like HIV, and drug-resistant strains of diseases including malaria, pneumonia, and tuberculosis, are spreading fast. Diseases formerly associated with the tropics are finding their way to temperate regions, and vice-versa.

In terms of gender-specific needs and interests, maternal death and illness statistics provide the most compelling evidence of the failure of health providers and development organisations to meet the often-discussed goals of safe motherhood and reproductive health. Currently, an estimated 585,000 women each year die as a result of childbearing (Panos 1998, 8). The lifetime risk to a woman of dying of pregnancy-related causes is one in 23 in

Africa, compared to one in 10,000 in developed countries (Doyal 1995, 11). 'About two-thirds of the world's women live in countries where per capita income is low and life expectancy relatively short, where the fertility rate continues to be high and a comparatively small percentage of the paid labour force is female, where class and gender inequalities in income and wealth continue to be very great, and the state provides few health and welfare services.' (ibid, 5)

Articles in this issue argue that two fundamental changes are needed if both women and men are to achieve better health. The first of these is to ensure equal access to all the resources that women and men need for healthy minds and bodies: not only to medical care, but to food, water, shelter, a source of income, and a sense of control over one's life. The second is to ensure that health services and resources enable women and men to meet *all* their health needs, including those that are gender-specific. Here, the issues that need to be addressed fall into three categories: the 'shape' (i.e. content) of health programmes; their quality; and their accessibility.

Health in a context of poverty: a gender analysis

In most sectors of development/social policy, gender analysis encourages us to focus on the cultural basis of difference between women and men, and consider how this shapes people's experience of poverty. This section takes a brief look at the impact of ideologies – which govern the decision-making power that we have, and the work we do – on women's and men's bodies and minds.

Reproductive work and health
Reproductive tasks – ranging from the work of childbearing and rearing to the care of the home – create particular health needs for women. Men's role in reproductive work is minimal in comparison to that of

women, and unequal power relations between the sexes means that they retain the ability in most households to define the terms on which women perform this work.

There is a strong onus on many women to 'give' children to their husbands, and, in a context of few economic options for women outside marriage, many women have little say in how many children they bear or at what intervals. In many societies, social and economic inequality between women and men is played out through regulating women's bodies, to ensure chastity before marriage and fidelity within it. 'Women's sexuality represents the interface between two of the most potent and insidious forms of oppression – gender and sexuality.' (Gordon and Kanstrup 1992, 29) Many women have little or no choice over when, where, and how they have sex, and hence no control over possible pregnancy or disease transmission. In her article on reproduction and infection among communities where HIV/AIDS is prevalent, Carolyn Baylies examines these issues. Women's experience of pregnancy, birth, and post-natal recuperation is likely to be shaped by the expectations of their families. In many places, decisions about childbirth and subsequent care for mother and baby are left to others. In their article, Judi Aubel *et al.* discuss the important role of older women in determining health outcomes for young mothers in Senegal.

In contexts of poverty and marginal-isation, women lose the innate biological advantage that they seem to have over men in terms of strength and longer life expectancy. Contrary to many popular gender stereotypes, there is considerable evidence to suggest that males are biologically weaker than females. Male embryos are more likely to miscarry during pregnancy, and, though more male babies are actually born than females, more of them die in infancy compared with female infants *who receive the same treatment* (Doyal 1995). However, if a woman lacks adequate nutrition, the means to control her fertility, and access to health care during pregnancy and birth, her biological advantage is offset by the toll that gender discrimination exacts on her. The work of caring for a family is arduous, time-consuming, and risky to women's health in poor communities everywhere. In the absence of water supplies, sanitation, and labour-saving devices, long hours spent carrying food and water and grinding grain cause back and neck injuries, while air pollution from cooking fires results in vulnerability to respiratory and eye diseases. One study of Colombian women living in poor households constructed over contaminated water showed how women, who stayed within the home to work, and collected water, were most at risk of cholera (Kitts and Roberts 1996).

Women provide an enormous amount of health care to family members. In addition to diagnosing and treating common illnesses, or deciding that a family member should seek external health care, women are typically responsible for the daily care of their families in terms of hygiene and sanitation. However, in some contexts they shoulder these responsibilities without having the requisite power to make significant decisions (for example, to take a child to hospital), or to make changes to unhealthy living conditions. In their article, Paule Simard and Maria De Koninck discuss women's role in water and sanitation provision in a peri-urban area of Bamako, Mali.

Production and health

In addition to their reproductive workload, women share with men considerable occupational health risks in the work they perform for production. However, a gender division of labour ensures that these risks are different for each sex, as well as varying in different locations. For example, women in rural areas who are involved in subsistence or cash-crop farming are likely either to have responsibility for different crops to men, or to have different tasks from men when tending the same crop.

Often, they are also required to balance productive activities with caring responsibilities. In some malarial areas, women weed and harvest crops before dawn, at the peak time for malaria transmission (Kitts and Roberts 1996).

In the past 20 years, women have become the preferred workforce in light industry and agricultural production for export. They face a new set of hazards from hazardous and exploitative working conditions. In addition to being unable to balance childbearing with their paid work (many are laid off if they are suspected of being pregnant), women working in low-paid jobs in factories experience a range of occupational health risks, ranging from eye strain from assembling small mechanical components, to poisoning from chemical dyes used in textile processing.

However, in most societies – both 'traditional' and modern – the most obviously risky or heavy productive tasks are heavily or exclusively male-dominated. Warfare, mine-work, and building and road construction are physically demanding and potentially dangerous to men. Men are vulnerable to injury and death in mining accidents, muscle strain in heavy labour of different kinds, and tropical diseases such as leishmaniasis (a group of parasitic diseases transmitted by sandflies) (Kitts and Roberts 1996). There is some evidence that men may also succumb to mental illness and depression brought on by the loss of the breadwinner role in societies where occupations seen as 'male' are dying. This is not confined to post-industrial societies; one study of rural Kenya where male livelihoods are in transition suggests: 'men feel inadequate, incompetent, insecure, inferior and persecuted.' (Silberschmidt 2000, 124)

Development perspectives on gender and health

What are the implications of the above gender analysis of health for development organisations whose vision of human development and wellbeing goes beyond a narrow understanding of development as growth in GNP and participation in the global 'free market'? In short, what are the links between gender, health, and poverty? Development workers have devoted considerable energy to examining the health impact of survival strategies of people in poverty, as they adapt to different economic conditions. Even where sustained economic growth has occurred, development along western lines has thus far failed to secure better health for women and men living in poverty in developing countries (any more than it has for those living in the 'South in the North'[1]).

Since the 1980s, development workers and researchers have also focused on shifts in donor priorities and government spending on the health sector. This area of enquiry has been of particular concern during the era of structural adjustment, in which many developing countries were required by international financial institutions to cut back on their public spending as a way of increasing the efficiency of their economies. Structural adjustment has had a dramatic impact on the wellbeing of people in poverty, and this impact has been different – and often worse – for women and girls. In the health sector, attempts to recover the cost of health care from 'consumers' are believed to serve the dual purpose of generating revenue and improving the efficiency of allocating services (Watkins 1998). In her article, Mohga Smith asserts the need for gender-sensitive means of monitoring and evaluation of health policies, to provide evidence that imposing user fees on patients further marginalises parts of the population, including women from poor communities, who cannot find the money to pay.

Other researchers in development have examined the links between education, women's 'empowerment', improvements in mother and child health, and reductions in family size. Some have stressed the fact that

'reduced access to education, information, and knowledge means that women are often poorly informed about health issues' (Kitts and Roberts 1996, 20), which affects women's ability to recognise illnesses, and either treat them at home or seek professional support. Others have argued, compellingly, that an excellent reason to address gender, education, and health together is that there is a causal link between better education, women having more power within the family, better family health, and reduced fertility. However, this link has been questioned. The fact that better-educated women tend to have healthier families and fewer children may be simply the result of the fact that both education and health care cost money in many places, and wealthier families are likely to choose to invest in both. Equally, reduced fertility, more spending on family health, and educating girls may not indicate women's greater autonomy so much as the fact that the male decision maker has led his family on a course of action which has practical benefits for women and children (Jeffery and Jeffery 1998). Speculation about the nature of the links between gender equity, health, and education – and about whether it is possible to develop a universal theory about this – continues.

Currently, the language of women's 'need' for essential resources including health care, which has been familiar to development and humanitarian workers for decades, is being replaced with a language of rights. This is due in part to the work of feminists in lobbying within their organisations and outside, and the outcomes of events including the series of UN Conferences on Women between 1975-95, and others. Huda Zurayk discusses the evolution of the reproductive health approach, which came to world attention during the 1994 UN International Conference on Population and Development in Cairo. This approach promoted an holistic vision of reproductive health that encompasses all aspects of women's health, rather than focusing narrowly on pregnancy, fertility control, and birth as processes which are isolated from the rest of women's lives. It also focuses on access to these services and the financing of them.

Since Cairo, the language of reproductive health and rights has passed into common usage among development organisations. However, while the women's movement focuses on women's human rights as an end in themselves, many development organisations see women's rights as an instrument which is needed to promote the development of wider society: '[I]f women do not have autonomy, they cannot make the health decisions that they are in the best position to make, they cannot see providers when they need to, they cannot use their family's limited resources in ways most likely to improve health.' (Stein 1997, 189) While this distinction may seem unimportant, it does potentially result in very different strategies. Huda Zurayk's article emphasises the importance of unpicking the differences between the agendas of different organis-ations. She argues that actors who used the language of population control prior to the Cairo conference in 1994 are now using the language of empowerment and rights, but remain uncommitted to the principles of promoting southern women's participation and self-determination. In turn, Colette Harris and Ines Smyth discuss the way in which reproductive health has been taken up by humanitarian relief organisations working with refugees. Reproductive health policies and programmes have begun to be implemented in refugee communities, and service-delivery has begun to be systematised. However, the participatory methods and emphasis on a holistic analysis that constitute cornerstones of the reproductive health approach present challenges to these organisations.

What prevents gender-equitable access to health?

This section considers some of the key concerns raised by health providers, community development workers, and women's health activists, about the quality and appropriateness of health programmes, and the degree of access that women have to them. Hilary Standing distinguishes between a 'women's health needs approach', signified by concern for the implications for women of gender differences in the experience of ill-health, and a 'gender inequality' approach, which focuses on the ways in which gender identities influence vulnerability to illness and determine one's ability to seek out health treatment. A women's health needs approach can result in two types of programme – focusing either on women-focused health interventions as a basic need, or on the cost-effectiveness to society of a focus on women's specific needs (Standing 1997).

In contrast, a gender inequality approach would focus on a health programme's social, economic, and political context, emphasising the need for analysis of male bias inside and outside all the institutions playing a part in delivering health care. Such an analysis could pinpoint ways in which health providers and the funding agencies which support them (both governmental and NGO) might work to improve the 'match' between health services and the women who need them.

Considering all health providers without bias in favour of medical models

Formal medical services are invariably inadequate to meet demand. Lack of infrastructure, equipment, drugs, and staff, dogs the medical services of many post-industrial countries, let alone those in developing countries. Economic austerity measures have increased this pressure during the past 15 years, and encouraged debate on extending the role of NGOs and the private sector in health service provision. Historically, non-state services have been provided in many developing countries (Standing 1997). However, many NGOs have focused their efforts on provision of preventative, as opposed to curative, health care (Smith, this issue).

Rather than visiting a hospital or clinic, many women and men depend instead on care at home (usually provided by women); on alternative forms of healing offered by 'traditional' health providers; or on pharmacies. This fact can be interpreted positively, as a vote of faith in non-formal health providers, in some contexts. For example, a woman with a low-risk pregnancy may prefer not to have a medicalised birth in hospital, while the different therapies offered by some traditional forms of healing may reflect the world view of service users more accurately than western models of sickness and health. In their article, Kate Butcher and Alice Welbourn discuss innovative ways of working with people with HIV and AIDS. They advocate a non-medicalised model of support and care that enables HIV-positive people to stay well for longer.

However, to some extent and in some cases, women's failure to use formal medical services indicates a failure to provide services that are sorely needed. The obvious example centres on pregnancy and birth.

Ensuring holistic and appropriate services

Maternal mortality statistics are among the clearest indicators of the marginalisation of women's gender-specific interests and needs. Worldwide, it is estimated that childbearing kills 585,000 women each year (Panos 1998, 8). Reducing the appalling death toll associated with childbearing is not just a matter of improving access to existing services. It is necessary to move beyond the narrow concerns of medical models of health, to consider *all* the causes of maternal mortality. This entails stepping

behind the immediate medical reasons for death, and addressing the social and economic contexts in which women become vulnerable to unsafe pregnancy.

In addition, the range of medical services offered needs to be appropriate. It is essential, in particular, that safe abortion is offered as a last resort when contraception fails women. Currently, it is estimated that 50 million abortions take place each year. Twenty million of these are unsafe, and about 95 per cent take place within developing countries. In Latin America, unsafe abortion is thought to cause 6,000 deaths each year, representing 25 per cent of the maternal mortality deaths for that region (ibid.). In their article, Deyanira González de León Aguirre and Deborah Billings discuss abortion in Mexico, in relation to safe motherhood and the attitudes of medical, religious, and governmental authorities.

The continuing failure to provide maternity services is particularly ironic in light of the fact that both health providers and women themselves tend to associate modern medical services for women *only* with issues of reproductive health (Kitts and Roberts 1996). Hence, non-reproductive health services tend to assume that women's concerns are the same as men's, and women are often deterred from seeking help as a result.

Ensuring affordability of essential drugs

There are also essential medical services which formal health providers fail to deliver for reasons of cost. The death rate from AIDS continues to rise across Africa, Asia, and Eastern Europe, while deaths in post-industrialised countries have plummeted since the mid-1990s due to the discovery and availability of anti-retroviral therapies. Recently, health activists from the South, in partnership with campaigners from international organisations, have challenged rules on international patents – to allow developing countries to produce cheap generic versions of these drugs – and lobbied the producers of these drugs to provide them at cost price. A recent court case brought by 39 major drug companies against the South African government was dropped. The drugs companies had taken the government to court in an attempt to block legislation giving it powers to import or manufacture cheap versions of brand-name drugs. In Brazil, by 1999, a similar supply strategy had decreased treatment costs by 70 per cent, enabling the health service to treat three times as many people for the same outlay, and saving tens of thousands of lives.[2]

Ensuring women's participation in planning services

The degree to which women participate in the planning, implementation, and manage-ment of health services – both formal and non-formal – has a direct impact on their value and relevance to users. Women have not been well-served by male-dominated medical research and development institutions and service providers. In their article, Rachel Tolhurst and Sally Theobald discuss their experience of 'mainstreaming' gender into health programmes, via a course in a UK university. The course offers skills-training on gender analysis to health professionals, to ensure that the control and treatment of infectious diseases integrates a gender perspective. This demands attention to the social context in which disease occurs, to the gap between women's health needs and the services they use, to the existence of alternative health services which may suit women better, and to the fact that women are not only potential users of health care services, but primary providers of care within their households.

Supporting home provision of care

As discussed above, women carry a huge burden of care for their families. In the absence of health services, or money to pay for them, women compensate by providing health care at home. In her article, Mohga Smith points out that debates about the impact of user-fees on communities in countries undergoing structural adjustment have focused on the impact on women of 'replacing' services formerly offered by the State. As Carolyn Baylies discusses in her article on HIV/AIDS in Zambia, while men who become sick or disabled tend to remain within the family home to be cared for, it is often a very different story when women are themselves ill. The fact that they are unable to perform their duties as wives and mothers, and the stigma attached to a woman with a sexually-transmitted disease, may lead to desertion or ostracism from the family. If a woman stays within her home, the responsibility for caring for her and for others often passes to her daughters, who end up sacrificing their chances of education. Emphasis should be on developing programmes that focus on alleviating the negative social and economic impact on women and men of disease and death which places new stresses on individuals and communities.

Conclusion

Good health is a – or perhaps *the* – critical asset on which human development and wellbeing depends. While good health itself can never be a right, in that it is the outcome of genetic and other biological processes as well as social and economic influences, all human beings have the right to quality health care. This right has not been realised in any country of the world to date. While developing countries grapple with the issue of financing health care systems which are groaning under the strain of reductions in public funding as they try to cope with existing and new diseases including HIV/AIDS, some post-industrialised countries are currently experiencing a resurgence in diseases associated with poverty. In the UK, for example, tuberculosis is increasing, having previously been virtually eradicated.

Health issues affect women and men very differently. They are also very different for populations in the South and North; and for the young and old. A holistic approach to health involves promoting the rights of women and men to equal access to the goods, services, and resources that they need in order to attain and sustain good health. This goes further than health services, drugs, or medical procedures; it is concerned with every aspect of human life.

Development organisations which have embraced a commitment to promoting gender equality have several different roles in promoting good health. In advocacy, their role is to ensure funding of appropriate and accessible health services, from governments and international bodies. This should include the development of effective medical treatments which are affordable to all, as a fundamental aspect of development and poverty eradication. Organisations working directly or in collaboration with communities on health issues should give attention to supporting the development of health services which have fully integrated a commitment to countering the economic and social factors that prevent marginalised parts of communities from enjoying good health. They should ensure the gender-sensitivity of health programmes, their good quality, and accessibility. Above all, women themselves need to be actively sought out and invited to participate in every level of health planning and delivery, to ensure their current contribution to achieving health for all is recognised, and their knowledge and commitment built on.

Notes

1 This refers to people living in poverty in more developed countries. People in poor communities in these countries often have worse health than those in rich communities within developing countries.

2 http://www.oxfam.org.uk/policy/papers/ctcbraz.htm

References

Doyal, L. (1995) *What Makes Women Sick: Gender and the Political Economy of Health*, Basingstoke: Macmillan.

Doyal, L. (2000) 'Gender equity in health: debates and dilemmas', *Social Science and Medicine*, 51(6).

El Bushra, J. (2000) 'Rethinking gender and development practice for the 21st century', *Gender and Development*, 8(1).

Gordon, G. and C. Kanstrup (1992) 'Sexuality: the missing link in women's health', *IDS Bulletin*, 23(1).

Jeffery, P. and R. Jeffery (1998) 'Silver bullet or passing fancy? Girls' schooling and population policy', in C. Jackson and R. Pearson, *Feminist Visions of Development*, London: Routledge.

Kitts, J. and J.H. Roberts (1996) *The Health Gap: Beyond Pregnancy and Reproduction*, Ottawa: IDRC.

Oxfam (2000) 'Fatal Side Effects: Medicine Patents Under the Microscope', Oxfam GB Briefing Paper. Available from Policy Department, Oxfam GB, 274 Banbury Road, Oxford OX2 7DZ.

Panos (1998) *Women's Health: Using Human Rights to Gain Reproductive Rights*, Panos Briefing no. 32, London: Panos.

Silberschmidt, M. (2000) *'Women forget that men are the masters': Gender Antagonism and Socio-Economic Change in Kisii District, Kenya*, Uppsala: The Nordic Africa Institute.

Standing, H. (1997) 'Gender and equity in health sector reform programmes: a review', *Health Policy and Planning*, 11(3).

Stein, J. (1997) *Empowerment and Women's Health: Theory, Methods and Practice*, London: Zed Books.

Watkins, K. (1998) 'Cost-recovery and Equity: the Case of Zimbabwe', paper prepared for WIDER.

The reproductive health of refugees:
lessons beyond ICPD

Colette Harris and Ines Smyth

The vulnerability of populations affected by conflict or environmental disasters was stressed at the International Conference on Population and Development (ICPD) held in Cairo in 1994. In particular, the high mortality and morbidity rates among refugees were emphasised. The ICPD and its Programme of Action have enabled a degree of consensus[1] to be reached on the importance of reproductive health and rights, including those of refugees and internally displaced people. Post-Cairo, some of the language and concerns of the ICPD Programme of Action are being brought into the initiatives of international agencies, including UN agencies and international NGOs. Reproductive health policies and programmes have started to be implemented in refugee communities, and service-delivery has begun to be systematised.[2] However, if the mistakes and abuses of past family-planning programmes are to be avoided, we need to integrate some critical insights from feminists working in the fields of health and anthropology. However, there are structural constraints within relief organisations and operations which need to be overcome if they are to benefit from such insights.

Refugees are, by definition, survivors, who use their personal and material resources to escape danger, persecution, and fear. They are also very vulnerable to threats to their physical well-being and identity, as well as to threats to their survival as a group (based on ethnic, religious, or other grounds). Their vulnerability needs to be understood in the context of the increase in global economic, social, and environmental insecurity over recent decades (Baud and Smyth 1997). The key elements of this 'new world disorder' are armed conflict, military actions, and the disappearance of old State structures, all of which have profound implications for biological reproduction (Pearson 1997, 12).

Data concerning the numbers of refugees in the world are notoriously unreliable. What is certain is that their numbers are on the increase. In the last few years, there has been an escalation in the numbers of those displaced by conflicts and by major natural disasters, as well as those forced to move by deliberate government policies. The International Federation of Red Cross and Red Crescent Societies (1995) reports that in 1985 there were 22 million refugees and internally displaced people, and that by 1995 their number had increased to 37 million. In 1998 alone, well over a million people in Central America, Bangladesh, Central Asia, and parts of Africa lost their homes in floods. Large numbers of refugees from Kosovo and East Timor have moved to neighbouring countries under extremely difficult conditions. It is impossible to assess how many of these people will be able to rebuild their homes and communities in the near future, and how many will continue to rely on relief agencies for help. Very long-term refugee camps now exist in a number of countries. There are also large numbers of people who have been displaced, but remain within the borders of their country of origin – at least 24 million, according to one estimate (Wulf 1994). Internally displaced people often flee their homes for the same reasons, and in the same circumstances, as those who have crossed national boundaries. However, the distinction in terminology means that they receive little recognition and help at international level, and thus, at times, may be substantially worse off than refugees who have left their country of origin.

The care of these refugee populations presents considerable challenges arising from the circumstances of extreme poverty, destitution, and insecurity in which most have to live, and the large numbers involved. They exist in a political vacuum, outside the 'normal' life of any country, stripped of political rights, and alienated from viable economic opportunities and from access to social provisioning. For large numbers of refugees, virtually the only services available – including health care – are those supplied by aid organisations. This applies not only to the first stages of emergency evacuation, but also to the succeeding stages which may continue, as has been noted above, for a very long time. Displacement is often considered a temporary situation, and the long-term solution is supposed to be repatriation to the place of origin or as near to it as possible. While a 'voluntary, safe return to their own countries' (Keen 1992) may well be the best solution to the refugees' problems, it is not always possible. Refugees represent a new type of population, rather than a temporary condition.

Refugees' health needs

The psychological and physical conditions in which refugees live may mean that they have greater need for health care and good nourishment than other citizens – either of the country of origin, or the host country. At present, the provision of health care for refugees is a long way from being adequate, and this is especially true with regard to reproductive health services. Women and children comprise a large proportion of the refugee and displaced population, at least in some contexts, and are sections of the populations with the largest health care needs.

Owing to the fact that interest in the reproductive health and rights of refugees is relatively recent, and the difficulties of carrying out studies at field level in certain situations, there is comparatively little research and information on the reproductive health status and needs of refugee women and men. It is often stated that at least 75 per cent of the world's refugee and displaced people are women and girls (Bandarage 1997), and that of these, 20 per cent are of reproductive age and 25 per cent are expectant mothers (Davidson 1995). The reproductive-health risks to which they are exposed are well known, but accurate information on the consequences is lacking. However, an impression can be gained from indirect statistical data. For example, maternal mortality in the countries between which refugees mostly move is up to 200 times higher than in Western nations (Poore 1995). Anecdotal evidence is sometimes used to claim very high fertility for women in refugee populations, but hard evidence for such a conclusion is often absent.

Whatever the statistics concerning the proportion of women among refugees, the conditions under which flight and resettlement take place hold greater dangers for women because of their disadvantaged position in gender relations, and their role in biological reproduction. Their ability to conceive, carry successful pregnancies to term and give birth to healthy babies, as well as their capacity to have sexual relations and lead reproductive lives free of violence and abuse, may all be affected. The situation may be further exacerbated by the breakdown of kinship ties or community networks on which women commonly rely during and after childbirth, or in times of illness. Similarly, women's traditional resources for contraception, abortion, and the like may be lost to them. Moreover, such situations are often marked by violence against women, including rape and forced sex in order to gain access to protection or the means of survival for themselves and their dependants. The possible consequences of sexually transmitted diseases and dangerous pregnancies are grave.

Lessons from Cairo and beyond

For several decades, feminists and other advocates working in the field of health and women's rights have been discussing issues related to reproductive health. The result has been a body of literature which has rehearsed many of the practical, theoretical, ethical, and political dilemmas concerning reproductive health.

This body of literature can be divided into two related categories, both of which could be of great use in developing health policies which take into account the specific circumstances of refugees, especially women. The first category comes out of the work of the international health movement, and is directly related to aspects of reproductive health. The second has emerged from the discipline of anthropology and, to a lesser extent, sociology. It is related to issues of cultural specificity and ways of working with local populations, and is not necessarily directly related to questions of reproductive health.

Feminist insights into reproductive health

As stated at the start of this article, the Plan of Action of the ICPD has provided a major impetus to interest in the reproductive health of refugees, and is also the source of the basic principles that are supposed to guide the provision of services. It is unanimously recognised that many of the positions taken by the Plan of Action are the result of the long-term influence of the work of feminist activists, academics, and health workers (Lassonde 1997).

A broader understanding of reproductive health
Among the most fundamental critical insights from feminist health advocates has been that reproductive rights are not limited to birth control, or to birth control plus mother-and-child health, sexually transmitted diseases, and HIV/AIDS. The concept encompasses many other aspects of health and well-being, including abortion rights, gynaecological health (including menstruation), issues of infertility (which may be a greater problem for some populations than the need for birth control), and sexual health (as well as violence). This expansion of the notion of reproductive health is a direct consequence of the critical stance that feminist and other health advocates have long taken in relation to population-control programmes (García Moreno and Claro 1994). Such programmes, they maintain, have focused on fertility reduction as the solution to what policy-makers perceive as the most pressing global problem: that of population growth, especially among the poor in developing countries. Sometimes they have added a concern for the containment of the growing pandemic of AIDS. Both these concerns have lent themselves to coercive treatment of populations (Hartmann 1987).

Another essential critique put forward by feminists is that reproductive health cannot be addressed merely as a medical matter. It cannot be separated from the conditions of poverty and insecurity in which many men and women in developing countries live. Such conditions often dictate reproductive and fertility behaviour, but they also determine access to adequate nutrition, sanitation, and health services. This understanding also helps to locate broader population issues in the context of economic growth and development. '...The population issue must be defined as the right to determine and make reproductive decisions in the context of fulfilling secure livelihoods, basic needs (including reproductive health) and political participation.' (Sen 1994)

Also central to feminist analysis is the idea that problems of reproductive health are related to gender-based power relations, which systematically disadvantage women and girls. This idea has several components. One is that, in most societies, women gain social status and position through their reproductive functions, so that their reproductive health has considerable repercussions for their overall existence (Gupta 1996). At the same time, many women in different locations enjoy little control over their reproductive behaviour and its outcome. In fact, women's sexuality and procreative functions are generally at the centre of far-reaching cultural norms. As a consequence, in many societies decisions about whether and when women should marry, with whom, when they should have sexual relations, and when and how many children they have, are controlled by spouses, other senior household members (for example, mothers-in-law), religious leaders, and policy-makers (Berer 1994). In particular, unmarried adolescent girls tend to be the focus of strict controls to guarantee not merely their virginity, but also a spotless reputation.

The emphasis of feminist health advocates on women and their reproductive health and rights does not mean that women are the only focus in these debates. It has been recognised for some time that men and adolescents of both sexes also have reproductive needs. Furthermore, these issues are not only the concern of people of reproductive age. Both older men, and post-menopausal women, have reproductive-health needs which should be acknowledged and taken into consideration.

Birth control and other medical provisions

Many of the relevant debates have concentrated largely on issues of birth control/family planning, as these were the major focus of the international community in the pre-Cairo era. Many studies have recorded the abusive character of fertility-control programmes (Dixon-Mueller 1993). Women in general, as well as minority groups under-represented in governments, have all too often been targeted for specific fertility-reduction programmes, including forced sterilisation (Hartmann 1987). At the same time, large numbers of people who might wish to use modern contraception do not have adequate access to affordable methods of their choice.

Coercive programmes have been shown to be very often ineffective, and even counterproductive. Research has indicated that countries such as India with the strongest population policies are not necessarily those that show the greatest reduction in fertility. Also, couples using modern methods of contraception do not necessarily have fewer children than those using traditional methods such as abstinence and breast-feeding (for example, Pearce 1995). The abusive practices of population-control policies have often made women less willing to use contraceptives (Ravindran 1993; Hartmann 1993). Therefore, groups of people who have been targeted by very strong population control programmes may be especially wary of contact with modern medicine and its practitioners, including modern methods of birth control.

The technology of these methods has also been a topic for considerably heated debate, particularly on the problems associated with hormonal and with provider-dependent long-acting contra-ceptives such as Norplant, Depo Provera and, more recently, vaccines (Hardon and Hayes 1998). The latter are attractive to international health-service providers and governments, since they have properties of effectiveness and ease of delivery (Sen and Snow 1994). On the other hand, many women have experienced negative side effects from long-acting hormonal contraceptives, including increased bleeding, headaches, weight-loss or gain, and even infertility (Panos 1994). Barrier methods, especially the female condom and the diaphragm, are insufficiently available, in great part because Western providers believe them to be unacceptable to local populations and also because they do not consider them effective enough (although HIV/AIDS has led to a re-evaluation of this position).

An important aspect of these debates, and the area in which there has been the most consensus, is the need to provide high-quality reproductive-health programmes. Since Cairo, the idea that these should not be limited to family planning but should instead include a wide range of reproductive health services is gradually becoming accepted. Furthermore, in relation to such services the concept of quality of care is often mentioned. This encompasses various components, the most important of which are choice of method; technical competence and good interpersonal skills of providers; full and informed consent in the choice of contraceptives; and appropriate constellations of services including mechanisms for follow-up (Bruce 1990).

Acknowledging the importance of cultural differences
Much can be learned from the work of feminist anthropologists, and others, who have been concerned with the need to acknowledge the cultural specificity of reproductive practices and beliefs and, as a consequence, the importance of sensitivity to cultural differences and needs at the micro-level.

Such analysts have shown that all too often it is assumed that all groups of women and men have similar reproductive-health needs. Individual country or culture-group studies have shown this to be untrue. Reproduction is an area particularly subject to cultural differences. In order for services to be relevant and acceptable, it is vital to situate reproductive health within people's real experience (Petchesky 1998). The tendency towards cultural generalisation is often unhelpful, and can be dangerous (Smith 1998). Such generalisations are often made in relation to religion and reproductive health. This tends particularly to be applied to Muslim populations, where a simplistic link between religion, women's subordination, and fertility is assumed. Any such relation is far from proven. It has been shown that religion is not necessarily a determining factor in the acceptance of contraceptives. For example, in Pakistan, 77.6 per cent of those surveyed in a USAID study said that they had not taken religion into consideration (Correa and Reichman 1994, 32). The indigenous cultural environment, together with the socio-economic and political circumstances of Muslims – as in the case of people professing other religions – are the main determinants of their reproductive behaviour, not their religion (see, for instance, criticisms of such approaches by Makhlouf 1991, 1994).

Crucially, for (feminist) health advocates, recognising the diversity of cultural attitudes to reproduction (as to other aspects of social life) is not synonymous with taking a relativist position, one which believes all cultural practices to be acceptable (Gasper 1996). On the contrary, they stress that within given cultures reproduction is a matter on which women, and other subordinate groups, are often oppressed and silenced.

In practice, this means that great cultural understanding and sensitivity are necessary both in order to assess needs, and in the provision of reproductive-health services. Such sensitivity is necessary to allow grassroots Southern women (but also boys, girls, and even men) to have a voice in all services provided for them, including those pertaining to reproductive behaviour and health. Furthermore, talking to the more educated, to male (or even female) leaders, and to others who present themselves as knowing and speaking for their communities, does not provide an adequate or full picture of the overall situation. The least educated and vocal minority ethnic and cultural groupings must be consulted directly too, in order to ensure that interventions meet their needs, and are effective.

A discourse which emphasises the legitimacy of specific cultural practice is also compatible with advocating the need for women to mobilise themselves to achieve increased reproductive rights (Petchesky 1998). Reproductive-health interventions should include ways through which women may in some cases be supported to understand what their rights are in this respect. For instance, a literacy course run in a rural area of Senegal introduced its female students to notions of reproductive rights. The students themselves subsequently thought out the implications of what they had learned for the practice of female genital mutilation, common in their communities. After some weeks of discussion among themselves, the women returned to the class and declared that hitherto they had not realised they had a right to do anything about such practices. They decided that from then on they would oppose female genital mutilation in their villages (personal communication from Bertrade Mbom, CUNY). While the need to incorporate local views and perspectives is recognised by all, in practice it remains difficult to realise.

The case of the WVV programme, Kenya

As an example of this point, we will use a study by Kathina (1998) of the Women Victims of Violence (WVV) programme in Dadaab camp, Kenya, to reflect on the difficulty of combining in practice a concern for the issues raised by women and health advocates with a true consideration for cultural differences.

Kathina's discussion makes it clear that the WVV programme in many ways attempted to address the needs of women refugees, and the concerns often raised by feminist health advocates. However, several aspects of the programme were based on pre-conceived and often Euro-centric views. The programme was based on the realisation that violence against women is high in refugee camps and puts them at significant risk. However, because a needs assessment was carried out in a superficial manner, it did not take into account the daily experiences of the most vulnerable women, but made assumptions about the nature of violence as well as the behaviour of women. Key assumptions were that the perpetrators of violence were necessarily 'outsiders' and that women spent their time exclusively within the (safe) confines of the camp. This bears considerable resemblance to the commonly held notion that women are safe within the private sphere, away from the dangers of the public domain (Sciortino and Smyth 1997). Thus, it was considered sufficient to build a fence around the camp to keep the violent (and violence) out. The fact that much of the violence came from within the camp, and that many attacks took place during women's daily forages outside the camp for firewood, was ignored.

Another problem was that the WVV programme seemed to have limited sensitivity to local cultures in the way it dealt with the women who had experienced rape. The Western-trained relief workers wished the women concerned to admit openly to having been raped, so that they could receive counselling. However, in the culture of the Somali women concerned, rape is a disgrace which marks a woman for life and makes it impossible for her to be accepted in her own community.

Women who acknowledge their situation publicly expose themselves to rejection by their families and communities and to the unwanted sexual attention of men. Even a woman's natal family cannot be seen to support her afterwards. In such circumstances, women may prefer to keep their experiences secret. Therefore, many of the women concerned felt they could no longer continue to live in Africa where everyone knew of their plight; so they applied to emigrate to the West. The programme officers were not sympathetic to this problem, seeing it as a mere ploy to gain refugee status in a Western country. The focus of the WVV programme displayed considerable sympathy for the issues that are a concern of women and health advocates, namely sexual violence in refugee situations. Nevertheless, it seems to have been very limited in its capacity to make significant improvements in refugee women's lives, and in fact it may have caused additional damage. In this, the programme is probably far from unique.

Unfortunately, as mentioned earlier, to date we have very few studies of other similar programmes, so much of our discussion inevitably remains speculative.

Obstacles to implementing effective reproductive-health programmes

It should be said that it is not easy to incorporate the sorts of lessons learned from (feminist) anthropological research into the actual programmes carried out in refugee situations. There are many reasons for this. The sheer scale and urgency of the problems, and especially the large numbers of people involved, often make them appear overwhelming. It also makes it difficult to work at the micro-level in a way which responds to the needs of so many diverse individuals and small groups. According to Lassonde (1997), the advantage of the notion of reproductive

health is that it is sufficiently flexible to allow the priorities and approaches of different – and differing – groups to be taken into account. However, she also stresses that there is a fundamental limitation: the fact that reproductive health '... is more a consensus-oriented idea than a standard-setting definition stipulating how programmes can be structured' (1997, 22).

In this section, we will highlight factors that, in combination with this limitation, may prevent policy-makers and practitioners from learning from feminist health and anthropological insights, and preclude the implementation of reproductive health programmes which truly reflect the needs and perceptions of different groups among the refugees themselves.

A factor which may militate against learning from the insights summarised earlier is that the multilateral and bilateral donors who fund most activities aimed at providing services to refugee populations may have agendas which differ greatly from their stated objectives. Behind a language which claims commitment to the well-being of refugees, including their reproductive health, other priorities may hide. Migrant and refugee populations are commonly blamed for environmental destruction, insecurity, and social problems. This may give rise to concerns for the political stability of particular geographical areas; neo-Malthusian[3] concerns about the growth of specific groups perceived to be unproductive, dependent, and/or politically volatile; or to concerns to limit the spread of disease among groups of people who are viewed as irresponsible.

Another factor is the personal capacities of policy-makers and implementers. No doubt a large number of middle- and upper-level officials involved both at policy- and decision-making levels and in practical work have a genuine commitment to improving the conditions under which refugees and other displaced people live. They may also have skills and expertise in technical and managerial fields, but may suffer from a lack of knowledge and understanding of crucial aspects of women's health, of anthropological information, and of gender and development issues. This applies also to staff working in NGOs.

In other words, there would appear to be a double dislocation within the international relief community. On the one hand is the dislocation between the policies stated at headquarters and in public pronouncements, and the programmes actually carried out on the ground. On the other hand, there is the dislocation between the commitment of the individuals working in relief agencies, genuinely trying to propagate helpful and positive approaches to refugee welfare, and their ability to realise such approaches in practice.

But such dislocations account for only some of the reasons that may prevent providers from meeting the needs of refugees. Many of the approaches to practical development interventions dominant among international organisations tend to be technocratic and to lack a holistic approach (Sen and Grown 1988). Reproductive health, as we have already pointed out, cannot be separated from other aspects of life. Research has shown that the attempt to deal with each aspect of refugee life separately is making it impossible to provide services that adequately correspond to needs. However, the international community has so far persisted in seeing such situations as technical problems with technical solutions. For example, one commentator discusses the likelihood that the provision of a largely grain-based diet to meat-eating, milk-drinking nomads within the camps has resulted in greatly increased levels of pre-eclampsia[4] (Wulf 1994).

Above all, the lack of sensitive, ongoing, and serious consultation of the mass of refugees, especially the most vulnerable – which include not only women but also children of both sexes – makes it impossible to tailor programmes to fit their needs.

In addition, at the level of programme and projects, a major problem is presented by the lack of appropriate information and training on the part of the project implementers. As stated earlier, the subject of reproductive health among refugee populations is closely related to some of the most complex and controversial cultural practices within all societies (Lee 1993). This means that extremely accurate information, and sensitivity in gathering it, is necessary when dealing with the provision of reproductive-health services. Staff of many agencies may not have the necessary skills and knowledge to ensure this. Even medical staff, otherwise interested and experienced, may not be equipped with specialised knowledge of reproductive health. The short length of contracts of staff working in relief programmes often means they have little opportunity to acquire additional necessary skills, such as relevant languages, cultural understanding of the locality, and gender-awareness. The lack of continuity in programmes and poor dissemination of relevant information and experience aggravate the situation.

Both UN agencies and NGOs are likely to suffer from such problems, although the staff of the latter may well have greater sensitivity to the issues involved. Local organisations and individuals are not immune to these problems. They are more likely to have a better knowledge of customs, languages, and needs. However, they may have little chance of influencing programmes in which they are engaged, because of the hierarchies often present in aid work which prevent local views and priorities from determining policies and programmes.

Overcoming the obstacles

The obstacles outlined in the previous section are not all surmountable by changes in tactics on the part of agencies and field workers. Some would require the total restructuring of the international aid community and its relationships with donors. However, there is much that could be done to improve the situation by concentrating on those problems which are easier to solve.

Working in line with participatory principles

The feminist and anthropological insights summarised above highlight the need for reproductive-health programmes to be designed in direct response to the needs and perspectives of refugees themselves, especially women (but also of men, children, and others of non-reproductive ages), and thus to be based on a sound knowledge and understanding of local cultural beliefs and practices. Such an approach may well reveal totally different requirements from those generally accepted. For instance, it may be that many refugee women are much more concerned about infertility and its causes than with controlling their fertility through contraception. Some populations may find abortion totally irrelevant or even abhorrent, while others expect abortion services as a matter of right.

The abundance of methods which have been devised for participatory and gender-sensitive planning could be put to use in working with refugees on designing their own programmes. These methodologies can help to ensure the participation of representatives of all groups involved. This includes women, children (or at least adolescents), old people, ethnic minorities, male and female representatives of all tribal and other minority groups concerned.

Such methods can only work if they are supported by knowledge and understanding. Major cultural and power differentials between various sub-groups of people may exist within apparently homogeneous cultural groupings. Furthermore, such sub-

groups may be in conflict with each other in the country of origin – even on opposite sides of a civil war. The resulting potential for conflict within settlements needs to be taken into account in all aspects of planning.

The understanding and use of such methods could have helped to avoid the errors of the WVV programme, discussed earlier. Consulting local women would have revealed the various *loci* of the violence against them, and this might have led to a different solution than that adopted. Similarly, an understanding of the rigidity of local cultural attitudes towards rape could have led to an attempt to help keep women's affairs private. Including local people at decision-making levels may help to reveal such attitudes more efficiently than an exclusive use of international staff.

Programme staff with experience of participatory methodologies should be recruited where possible. Anthropologists – especially those trained in the more sensitive methodologies, such as feminist anthropology – would be an invaluable source of knowledge and advice. Staff drawn from the population served, especially in higher positions, would provide relevant knowledge and insights. On the other hand, it is important to be sensitive to local politics and divides, and to avoid privileging certain cultural, religious, or ethnic groups. The recruitment of female staff does not necessarily render programmes more sensitive to the needs of female refugees, but it can facilitate communication with refugee women (especially on sensitive topics) as well as offering them employment opportunities.

Implementing programmes with women and refugee organisations

Many of the programmes aiming to provide reproductive-health services for refugees would benefit from being implemented in collaboration with, or at least with the advice of, women and refugee organisations. Among the advantages offered by these agencies is their ability to work more closely with communities, and with a better understanding of local cultures and needs than large international or government institutions. This approach can also improve the sustainability of programmes, as local civil society organisations will still be there when an externally initiated programme is completed.

It is also important to learn from existing innovative programmes and, when appropriate, transfer their lessons to other situations. From 1997, the University of Zimbabwe (University of Zimbabwe Project Support Group Reproductive Rights and Health Partnerships) sponsored one such programme, with community organisations in southern Africa. It provides contraceptives and information on birth control to large numbers of people with minimum costs, using local grassroots organisational networks.

The acquisition of knowledge and understanding of local circumstances and of the insights and theories discussed above can be facilitated by closer links with the academic community. For example, Moi University in Nairobi and the University of Amsterdam have the subject under consideration, while others, such as the London School of Hygiene and Tropical Medicine, have been running relevant courses for years.

Conclusion

We have identified a number of obstacles to the translation into effective action of the many lessons that emerge from feminist and anthropological approaches to reproductive health and rights. We also pointed out that the scarcity of research and accurate information on the reproductive practices of displaced people, and of existing policies and programmes, limits our understanding of both.

We have suggested that the adoption of participatory methodologies, collaboration with and direct involvement of refugee institutions and individuals, improvements in skills and understanding, and even changes in recruitment practices would all facilitate the implementation of services that reflect genuine needs and perspectives of the beneficiaries. These changes would go some way to counterbalance the vulnerability of displaced people, by enabling them to contribute more directly to interventions affecting their reproductive health.

A more fundamental change is, however, necessary. Recently, the major institutions active in the field of reproductive health have agreed on the need to commit resources to its promotion. However, this general agreement does little to set standards for the quality of the services provided. This may make it easy for organisations involved in humanitarian interventions to carry out activities which do not necessarily match their language. A crucial step towards programmes which effectively address the many reproductive-health needs and problems of refugee populations is that such organisations should be more explicit in their purpose and coherent in their practices, and thus more accountable to those they claim to serve. It is this accountability which, again, would make refugees and internally displaced people less vulnerable, not only in matters concerning their reproductive health but in all processes and decisions which affect their lives.

Colette Harris is Programme Director for Women in Development in the Office of International Research and Development at Virginia Tech University, 1060 Litton Reaves Hall, Blacksburg, VA 24061-0334, USA.
E-mail: harriscolette@hotmail.com

Ines Smyth is a Policy Adviser for Oxfam GB, 274 Banbury Road, Oxford OX2 7DZ.
E-mail: ismyth@oxfam.org.uk

This article is an edited version of a longer chapter in the forthcoming book Managing Reproductive Life: Cross Cultural Themes in Fertility and Sexuality, *edited by Soraya Tremayne. The book will be published in Autumn 2001 by Berghahn Books, 3 Newtec Place, Magdalen Road, Oxford OX4 1RE, UK. E-mail: editorialUK@berghahnbooks.com*

Notes

1 There are doubts about the strength of this consensus, strongly differing views on the subjects of reproduction, sexuality, and population issues mentioned earlier.

2 Recent initiatives include: the establishment of an inter-agency working group (IAWG), the publication of a field manual for relief organisations, and the creation of UNHCR's guidelines on the provision of services in reproductive health for refugees.

3 Malthus stressed that population growth resulted in famine and destitution. More modern versions of similar ideas argue that the earth has limited capacities to support its inhabitants, and environmental degradation is attributed mainly to population pressures.

4 Pre-eclampsia (formerly known as toxaemia) is a complication of pregnancy that can affect both the woman and the foetus.

References

Bandarage, A. (1997) *Women, Population and Global Crisis*, London: Zed Books.

Baud, I. and I. Smyth (1997) 'Searching for security: women's responses to economic transformations', in I. Baud and I. Smyth (eds), *Searching for Security: Women's Responses to Economic Transformations*, London: Routledge.

Berer, M. (1994) 'Motherhood, fatherhood and fertility: for women who do and women who don't want to have children', *Reproductive Health Matters*, 4: 6-11.

Bruce, J. (1990) 'Fundamental elements of the quality of care: a simple framework', *Studies in Family Planning*, 21.

Correa, S. and R. Reichman (1994) *Population and Reproductive Rights: Feminist Perspectives from the South*, London and New Jersey: Zed Books.

Davidson, S. with L. Lush (1995) 'What is reproductive health care?' *Refugee Participation Network*, 20: 4-8.

DFID (1997) Report on DFID Sponsored Research Workshop on Healthcare in Unstable Situations, Centre for International Child Health, Institute of Child Health, London.

Dixon-Mueller (1993) *Population Policy and Women's Rights: Transforming Reproductive Choice*, Westpoint: Praeger.

García Moreno, C. and A. Claro (1994) 'Challenges from the women's health movement: women's rights versus population control', in G. Sen, A. Germain, and L. C. Chen (eds) *Population Policies Reconsidered: Health, Empowerment and Rights*, New York: IWHC.

Gasper, D. (1996) 'Culture and development ethics: needs, women's rights and western theories', *Development and Change*, 27: 628-59.

Gupta, J.A. (1996) 'New Freedoms, New Dependencies: New Reproductive Technologies, Women's Health and Autonomy', PhD Thesis, Leiden University.

Hardon, A. and E. Hayes (eds) (1998) *Reproductive Rights in Practice: A Feminist Report on Quality of Care*, London: Zed Books.

Hartmann, B. (1987) *Reproductive Rights and Wrongs: The Global Politics of Population Control and Contraceptive Choice*, New York: Harper and Row.

Hartmann, B. (1993) 'The present politics of population and reproductive rights', *Women's Global Network for Reproductive Rights Newsletter*, 43: 1-3.

International Federation of Red Cross and

Red Crescent Societies (1996) *World Disasters Report 1996*, Oxford: Oxford University Press.

Kathina, Monica (1998) 'A Pilot Study of Refugee Camps in Kenya', unpublished paper for Research Project on Reproductive Health in Post-Crisis Situations in Africa, University of Amsterdam, NL.

Keen, D. (1992) *Refugees: Rationing the Right to Life*, London: Zed Books.

Lassonde, L. (1997) *Coping with Population Challenges*, London: Earthscan.

Lee, R. (1993) *Doing Research on Sensitive Topics*, London: Sage.

Makhlouf, O. C. (1991) *Women, Islam and Population: is the Triangle Fateful?*, Working Paper Series no 6, Harvard School of Public Health, Harvard Center for Population and Development Studies.

Makhlouf, O. C. (1994) 'Religious doctrine, state ideology, and reproductive options in Islam', in Sen and Snow (eds).

Panos (1994) *Private Decisions, Public Debates: Women, Reproduction and Population*, London: Panos.

Pearce, T. O. (1995) 'Women's reproductive practices and biomedicine: cultural conflicts and transformations in Nigeria', in F. D. Ginsberg and R. Rapp (eds), *Conceiving the New World Order: The Global Politics of Reproduction*, Berkeley: University of California Press.

Pearson, R. (1997) 'Global change and insecurity: are women the problem or the solution?', in I. Baud and I. Smyth (eds), *Searching for Security: Women's Responses to Economic Transformations*, London: Routledge.

Petchesky, R. P. and K. Judd, (eds) (1998) *Negotiating Reproductive Rights: Women's Perspectives Across Countries and Cultures*, London: Zed Books.

Poore, P. (1995) 'Delivering reproductive health care', *Refugee Participation Network*, 20: 16-20.

Ravindran, S. (1993) 'The politics of women', *Population and Development in India*, 8(3): 27-42.

Sciortiono, R. and I. Smyth (1997) 'The triumph of violence: the denial of domestic violence in Java', *Austrian Journal of Development Studies*, XIII(3): 299-319.

Sen, G. (1994) 'Development, population, and the environment: a search for balance', in G. Sen, A. Germaine, and L. C. Chen (eds), *Population Policies Reconsidered: Health, Empowerment and Rights*, New York: IWHC.

Sen, G. and K. Grown (1988) *Development, Crises and Alternative Visions*, London: Earthscan.

Sen, G. and R. Snow (1994) *Power and Decision: The Social Control of Reproduction*, Harvard Series on Population and International Health, Cambridge MA: Harvard University Press.

Shankar Sing, J. (1998) *Creating a New Consensus: The International Conference on Population and Development*, London: Earthscan.

Smith, S. (1998) 'Gender, Culture and Development: AGRA East Workshop Report', Hanoi: Oxfam.

UN (1994) *Programme of Action of the International Conference on Population and Development*, Report of the International Conference on Population and Development (Cairo, 5-13 September 1994), Section 7.2.

Wulf, D. (1994) *Refugee Women and Reproductive Health Care*, New York: Women's Commission for Refugee Women and Children.

The meaning of reproductive health for developing countries:

the case of the Middle East

Huda Zurayk

The International Conference on Population and Development (ICPD), held in Cairo in 1994, marked a major change for population and health policies in developing countries by recognising a new 'reproductive health' approach, and incorporating it into its Programme of Action. The new approach moved the focus of population policy from population growth and its consequences at a societal level, to individual health and wellbeing, and satisfaction of reproductive intentions. This article discusses the progress of population and health professionals in integrating the concept into their work, and offers some pointers in relation to the interests and needs of women in the Middle East region.

There have been many attempts to define the concept of reproductive health by population and health professionals, both preceding and following ICPD. One of the first definitions to appear came from a Reproductive Health Working Group (RHWG) in the Middle East region that was established in 1988, as part of a programme of the Population Council regional office in Cairo. The RHWG brought a multi-disciplinary perspective to its work of contributing to an improvement in reproductive health in the Middle East, taking into account women's social situation and the cultural context of the region. It has since grown in activity and membership and includes researchers from many countries of the region, with affiliated country teams in Egypt, Jordan, Lebanon, and Palestine. (De Jong 1999)

It should be noted that these widely used definitions of reproductive health recognise four dimensions of the concept, namely: reproductive choice, physical health of women and children, psychological health and well-being, and access to services. While there is implicit recognition in these definitions of the importance of all four dimensions, each dimension emphasises a different element of reproductive health.

Developing the concept

The reproductive health approach had started to develop some years previously, in the late 1980s, when it became clear that a holistic approach to understanding the process of reproduction was needed to guide population and health policies in developing countries. The approach was a marked contrast to those of the 1960s and 1970s, when the focus was on population policies that stressed fertility control and the need to slow population growth in developing countries. Population policies promoted family planning to achieve this end. In the early 1980s, the focus was expanded to include the concept of 'safe motherhood', in recognition of the continuing tragedy of maternal mortality (deaths of women during the period of pregnancy and delivery) in developing countries. Significant as this approach is in its concern with healthy childbearing, it does not extend its focus beyond periods of childbearing to address wider issues of women's reproductive rights and women's perspectives.

At ICPD, the concept of reproductive health became a central concern for health policy-makers and international development planners. This came about largely as a result of advocacy activities in the international arena, by the feminist movement and women's health advocates (McIntosh and Finkle 1995), who felt that women bear the greater burden of ill-health from childbearing while they also suffer from a lack of control over their bodies, their fertility, and their health (Ravindran 1995). They called for the attention of health policy-makers to be turned to the aim of ensuring healthy reproduction in all its facets, for all women, encapsulated in the concept of women's reproductive health.

Debates on reproductive health

Since ICPD, the reproductive health approach has been adopted by all UN organisations, and is being implemented in numerous countries. Unfortunately, the implementation of this approach has not embodied its liberating underlying ideology, which recognises the realities of women's lives and advances the necessity of the empowerment of women to achieve their reproductive rights (Zurayk 1999). Moreover, there is still some doubt about the appropriateness and impact of this approach, particularly among professionals in the population movement. They feel that the approach is diverting attention and resources from fertility control – which they consider a priority area of population policy – to a much wider concern with women's health.

The reproductive health approach must be given time and the chance to prove its usefulness. In adopting a wider perspective on reproduction, it aims to realise the rights of couples – women and men alike – to reproductive choice, as well as to healthy reproduction. These two goals, linked together and seen within the underlying social context, are more likely to be achieved than the top-down goal of fertility control.

The reproductive health approach has a great potential for success, yet achieving its goals in developing countries depends on the extent to which it is sensitive to the specific situations in which women find themselves in these countries. The early history of the concept, and in particular the fact that it was brought to the international arena through the efforts of the (largely western) feminist movement, means that more guidance from developing countries is needed if the concept is to develop further and be of use to women in different contexts.

Below, I discuss three contexts for reproductive health in developing countries, which in my view should be borne in mind by health policy-makers and planners in international and national contexts, if the reproductive health approach is to be brought to full fruition.

Contexts of reproductive health

Lifecycles and gender relations

As population policy was mainly concerned with fertility control, it centred its attention on women aged 15 to 45 and therefore capable of reproduction. As the reproductive health approach emerged, it kept its focus primarily on women in this age group, while transforming its concern from how to control fertility to how to achieve healthy reproduction. It became clear that a more holistic approach to reproduction would necessitate the incorporation of other age groups and men in its concern. At least three justifications can be made for widening the perspective of the reproductive health approach in this way.

I will illustrate these justifications from the experience of the Giza Morbidity Study in Egypt, in which I was a major participant. This study was conducted in two villages close to Cairo between 1989 and 1990 by a sub-group of the RHWG composed of social, medical, and public health scientists. The main objectives of the study were to explore the extent to which the health implications of reproduction influenced women's morbidity and quality of life, and to show the interaction of the social conditions of women's lives with their reproductive health. The study approached a random sample of women to interview them in their homes and to undertake a gynaecological examination in the village health centre. Ninety-two per cent of the women approached responded, yielding a sample size of 509 women. In-depth qualitative research was also undertaken with some women, and with key informants in the villages. The results of this study are extremely revealing (Khattab 1992; Khattab, Younis, and Zurayk 1999).

In order to be effective, the reproductive health approach must expand its concern to women of all ages: those preparing for reproduction and those in reproductive age groups, as well as those who are beyond reproduction. While it is true that reproduction occurs among women in the 15-45 age group, attaining the goal of healthy reproduction for all entails healthy preparation for reproduction in younger age groups. It is particularly important that girls and young women in developing countries receive sufficient nutrition in their early years. They must also have a good level of education and access to information, to prepare them for having children. For women beyond 45, reproduction may have ended, but the

health consequences of having borne children, particularly for those women with high levels of fertility, can be serious. In the study we conducted in Egypt, it was revealed that women over 65 suffer from a multiplicity of conditions related to reproduction, such as genital prolapse, hypertension, urinary tract problems, and obesity (Khattab, Younis, and Zurayk 1999).

If we expand the concern of the reproductive health approach to all age groups, it becomes easier for us to address the implications of the fact that reproduction occurs within the family, and is thus influenced by family conditions and by the power relations within families. Unequal power relations exist between men and women, and attention must be given to improving women's decision making power related to reproduction and reproductive health care. In addition, unequal power relations often exist between older women and younger women. This produces a level of complexity in family dynamics that must be taken into account in an analysis of the process of reproduction and of reproductive health care.

The reproductive health approach must not neglect men. Men are not only approximately half the population, but are also primary decision makers at all levels of society. Men are active players in the reproductive health context. They influence fertility decisions, the extent to which contraceptive methods are used, and whether or not women have access to health care (Khattab 1992). Their reproductive behaviour can endanger not only themselves, but also their partners; this is particularly true regarding sexually transmitted diseases and HIV/AIDS. Proponents of the reproductive health approach have gradually absorbed the need to incorporate men into programmes, and have moved to do so. However, compared with the long history of such programmes of working with women, there is a need to accumulate research and field experiences in developing countries that can help to guide this process. Above all, as we expand the concern of the reproductive health approach to include men, it is important to retain a central concern in gender analysis: the power imbalance between men and women and the consequences of that imbalance on women's lives and health (Cottingham and Myntti forthcoming 2002).

Understandings of health in context

In western countries, ill-health is mainly understood and addressed within a biomedical context, so that health is widely understood to be a medical issue. In developing countries, different systems for understanding health and disease may be very widely accepted. There is a need to broaden the perspective of health providers in developing countries in terms of their awareness of the variety of approaches to ill-health and of the influence of the social context (particularly poverty) on health. Unfortunately, the training of health providers in developing countries is often modelled on training systems in western countries. Not only do providers then adopt the biomedical approach to recognition and treatment of ill-health conditions, but they may also neglect factors in the social context that play a major role in the production of health and ill-health in developing countries.

For example, in many communities in Middle Eastern countries, women may consider that symptoms they experience, such as vaginal discharge and the heaviness they may feel because of the prolapse of reproductive organs, are a 'normal' consequence of their reproductive function, because so many women around them experience these symptoms (Khattab, Younis, and Zurayk 1999). If a reproductive health clinic serving these women does not include outreach services and health education activities, they may not become aware of the seriousness of the symptoms

they are experiencing, and will not come to the clinics for treatment.

Another example centres on the advice given by a medical doctor to a woman in our study population in Giza, Egypt, as she was leaving hospital after undergoing a hysterectomy. She was told by the physician in charge that she should eat well and rest for the coming month. As soon as the woman returned to her house in the village there was pressure on her to return to work at home and in the fields, being a precious resource to a poor family. How could she refuse? And how could she eat well, placing herself above her children and husband within the limited resources this family had for food? She was back in hospital within a week (Khattab 1992). Surely the physician could have made an effort to understand her circumstances, to ask to explain her medical situation and its implications to her husband, and perhaps to develop with both of them clearer guidelines on what she should and should not do, to support her period of recovery?

The cultural context

As indicated above, the reproductive health approach emerged at ICPD in 1994 largely as a result of the efforts of women in the western feminist movement. Women from the developing world who participated were mainly situated within the networks created by organisations in that movement (Al Baz and Zurayk 1996). One wonders, therefore, whether the issues given centre stage at the conference, such as abortion, female circumcision, and emerging family forms, are really top priority in the minds of women in developing countries, even the activists among them (Zurayk 1999). In setting priorities as the reproductive health approach continues to develop, there should be more active and independent participation of women in developing countries, particularly around sensitive issues.

To illustrate this point, there are several concepts in reproductive health that may have special cultural meaning within the

Middle East region, and should therefore be taken into account by reproductive health policy-makers in that region. For example, the world has risen against the practice of female circumcision, describing it as female genital mutilation. While recognising the urgent need to end this practice, particularly in its more severe form, one wonders at the publicity and the priority given to this practice by the West, in the face of so many other equally serious problems for girls and young women in the Middle East. Low school enrolment and high drop-out rates for girls in many countries in our region are catastrophic realities which need attention, for example. It is also important to understand why men demand the practice of circumcision for their daughters, and why women also seek it for their daughters despite having suffered it themselves, before we can intervene sensitively and effectively to end the practice.

To return to the issue of population, 'excess fertility' is another concept that has been labelled internationally as a health problem, but that has arguably resulted from a different concern: namely, the high rate of population growth in developing countries. While recognising the possible health effects on mothers and on children of a large number of births combined with short birth intervals, there is also a need to recognise that having a large number of children can bring happiness and well-being to couples, particularly in poor communities. This is not to argue for high fertility, but to call for cultural sensitivity in not describing it as a health problem. Families may choose high fertility for their psychological well-being (which is certainly part of health), and achieve it in a healthy manner. The emphasis should not be on the large number of children but on whether it is possible to achieve good levels of reproductive health within given resources.

Finally, there is the concept of 'consensual sex'. A concern has emerged, as part of the reproductive health approach, with 'healthy sexuality' (Tsui, Wasserheit, and Haaga 1997). In defining what this is, western frameworks largely influence what is to be considered healthy behaviour. Should every sexual act be consented to? If so, how can that be understood within marriages where the choice of the husband has not been subject to consent by the woman? As we attempt to come up with definitions of healthy sexuality, and of other healthy states that might be taken by health-care providers as a basis for health programmes, there is a need to recognise that the meaning of some key concepts may vary across cultures. In a concern for healthy sexuality, for example, one could begin to address violations to norms that are common across cultures, such as sexual violence and sexual exploitation of children (Tsui, Wasserheit, and Haaga 1997). This would prepare the environment for dealing with other issues such as consensual sex which are not as common a concern across cultures.

Conclusion

The objective of this article has been to give voice to a view from the Middle East, on the continuing development of the reproductive health approach. I have argued that this approach should be expanded beyond women of reproductive age to include younger and older women and also men, while incorporating at the same time the dynamic power relations related to age and gender in societies of the developing world. I have also argued for a wider perspective to be given to the meaning of health, which tends to be equated with a biomedical approach. What is needed is a holistic approach, which takes into account the perception of women and men about their health, and the influence of their social realities on the production of health and ill-health. This will shape the nature of the provision of reproductive health care. Finally, I have argued for more cultural sensitivity in understanding concepts within the reproductive health approach that may have cross-cultural variations in meaning.

Huda Zurayk is Professor of Biostatistics and Dean of the Faculty of Health Sciences (FHS) of the American University of Beirut (AUB). Before that, she worked as Senior Associate in the Population Council Cairo Office (1988-98), where she co-ordinated the regional Reproductive Health Working Group (RHWG). Postal address: c/o The Faculty of Health Sciences, American University of Beirut, Beirut, Lebanon.
E-mail: hzurayk@aub.edu.lb

References

Al Baz and H. Zurayk (1996) 'Forum on Women's Conference in Beijing: background and objectives', *Al Mustaqbal Al Arabi:* 104, 102, 204

Cottingham, J. and C. Myntti (forthcoming 2002) 'Reproductive health: conceptual mapping and evidence', in G. Sen, A. George, and P. Ostlin (eds), *Engendering International Health: The Challenge of Equity,* Chicago: MIT Press.

de Jong, J. (1999) 'Foreword', in H. Khattab, N. Younis, and H. Zurayk, *Women, Reproduction, and Health in Rural Egypt,* Cairo: The American University in Cairo Press.

Fathalla, M.F. (1991) 'Reproductive health: a global overview', *Annals of the New York Academy of Sciences,* I:1-10.

Khattab, H. (1992) *The Silent Endurance: Social Conditions of Women's Reproductive Health in Rural Egypt,* Amman: UNICEF; Cairo: The Population Council.

Khattab, H., Younis, N., and H. Zurayk (1999) *Women, Reproduction, and Health in Rural Egypt,* Cairo: The American University in Cairo Press.

Klugman, B. (1996) 'ICPD plan of action; its ideological effects', *Health and Transition Review,* 6(1):98-100.

McIntosh, A. and J. Finkle (1995) 'The Cairo conference on population and development: a new paradigm?', *Population and Development Review,* 21(2):223-60.

Ravindran, S. (1995) 'Women's health policies: organising for change', *Reproductive Health Matters,* 6:7-11.

Chowdhury, S., Egero, B., Myntti, C., and H. Rees (1996) 'Sexual and Reproductive Health: The Challenge for Research', discussion paper, Swedish International Development Cooperation Agency and World Health Organization.

Tsui, A.O., Wasserheit, J.N., and J.G. Haaga (eds) (1997) *Reproductive Health in Developing Countries Expanding Dimensions, Building Solutions,* USNAS Panel on Reproductive Health, Washington DC: National Academy Press.

United Nations (1994) *Program of Action of the 1994 International Conference on Population and Development,* A/CONF. 171/13, reprinted in *Population and Development Review,* 21(1):187-213 (chapters 1-VIII) and 21(2):437-61 (chapters IX-XVI).

Zurayk, H. (1988) 'A framework of ideas for development of a research agenda for the working group on reproductive health', a paper presented at the first meeting of the Working Groups of the Special Program of Research and Technical Consultation on Family Resources, Child Survival, and Reproductive Health, Cairo: The Population Council.

Zurayk, H. (1999) 'Reproductive health and population policy: a review and a look ahead', in A.I. Mundigo (ed.), *Reproductive Health: Program and Policy Changes Post-Cairo,* Belgium: International Union for the Scientific Study of Population.

Environment, living spaces, and health:
compound-organisation practices in a Bamako squatter settlement, Mali

Paule Simard and Maria De Koninck

This article is based on a study conducted in Samé, a squatter settlement on the outskirts of Bamako, capital of Mali. The objective was to observe how individuals and their families ensure health and well-being through organising everyday life in their compounds (the basic housing unit in African cities). The compound is mainly a female living and working space, since women are responsible for the majority of household-maintenance tasks, child care, and care of adults. Attention was focused particularly on the connection between women's responsibilities and their decision-making power in managing the compound. In addition, the social relationships between landlords and tenants were studied.

Researchers working within a development context have only relatively recently become interested in the urban environment (Stren and McCarney 1992). The Brundtland Report (1987) first stimulated widespread attention to the problems of large cities in the developing world. However, most researchers have concentrated their efforts mainly on problems of urban growth, inadequate health infrastructures, and the proliferation of spontaneous housing brought about by low standards of living and by meagre government resources (Stren 1992; Antoine *et al.* 1987). In general, research on the urban environment has tended to focus on the infrastructure, rather than on people's daily living conditions, or their behaviour and practices.

Nonetheless, a focus on everyday life in urban areas does exist. It has been explored mainly within the 'women, environment, and development' approach in studies of the rural environment, where women's impact on nature is most evident (Momsen and Kinnaird 1993; Sontheimer 1991; Monimart 1989). These studies are informed by the feminist belief that daily life needs to be examined if researchers are to understand social relations, including gender relations (Smith 1987; Dagenais 1994). So far, however, women in African urban areas have attracted relatively little attention from researchers. When they have, it has been mainly from the perspective of examining their access to decent housing, and their role in supplying water and in managing liquid and solid waste – that is, the way in which women deal with whatever resources they have access to (Moser and Peake 1987). Few studies have focused on urban women's strategies for organising work and activities, or managing their own private environment. Yet insights into such practices can be helpful in understanding women's conceptions of the urban environment and, more fundamentally, of health and well-being.

Accordingly this article considers the urban environment from a development perspective, rather than as an environmental issue, in agreement with the following statement: 'Development needs must take precedence over direct environ-mental needs, insofar as poverty is the major linking factor between the economic system and its human and environmental effects' (Stren and McCarney 1992, 26). The research study on which the article draws focused on the organisation of a squatter settlement in Bamako, Mali, and aimed to test the hypothesis that in Sahelian cities (and specifically in squatter settlements) gender relations and property relations are most significant in ensuring decent living conditions and good health among family members.[1] The study's objective was to identify the women residents' conceptions of health, and their daily practices to promote it, through the organisation and maintenance of their compound. We also sought a better understanding of how women's responsibilities for the health of family members was related to their decision-making power.[2]

In the following sections, we first discuss the environment in which the study took place, and the organisation of daily life in a compound, before focusing on the organisation and maintenance of the compound itself. After that, we go on to identify certain conceptions of health as they were communicated to us by members of the community in the Bamako settlement, in order to suggest connections between such conceptions and people's practices.

Living in Samé

The neighbourhood of Samé initially attracted our interest because an urban development project was already underway.[3] We therefore reasoned that we would be able to study a range of environmental issues in the area: not only land-management practices in the compounds, but also the differing stakes held by members of the community in restoring the neighbourhood (Geneau and

Simard 1995), and the impact of involvement in community associations on women's conceptions of the environment (Beauregard 1996).

In 1987, Bamako's population was 658,275 (the estimate for 1997 is 1.2 million), which represents 8.62 per cent of the national population and 22 per cent of the urban population of Mali (figures estimated to have increased to 12.9 per cent and 55 per cent respectively in 1997).[4] Bamako was founded by the French during the colonial era, to consolidate their hold on the interior of Africa. It developed around a colonial quarter and central 'native' quarters. Because Bamako was built on a plain stretching along both banks of the Niger river, few obstacles limited its expansion, and the city continues to grow. It now covers approximately 100 square kilometres, absorbing neighbouring villages, which have rapidly been transformed into squatter settlements (Diarra 1992). In 1987, 40 per cent of Bamako's population lived in squatter settlements.

The neighbourhood of Samé is located in the extreme north-west of Bamako, and is one of the only neighbourhoods on hilly land, which thereby curbs its growth. Samé is isolated as a result of its unusual geography, although it is closer to the city centre (approximately 5km) than the other squatter settlements on the urban periphery (more than 10km). Samé developed during the 1950s, when the inhabitants of the neighbouring village of Koulininko, followed by migrants from other Bamako districts, settled in Samé. The area now has a population of about 3000, divided among 180 compounds (Schatz and Muller 1991). The present-day inhabitants of Samé do not have legal ownership of the land, in the sense that they hold no land titles. The term 'owner' is therefore used here in an informal sense to refer to a person who has 'bought' a lot from a customary owner or from another intermediary, and has built a house on it.[5]

There is a stream in the neighbourhood; its banks have been planted with mango trees, to provide shade and cooler air. However, despite the advantages of this, the area is dilapidated, and accumulated garbage and waste water constitute a threat to the health and safety of both children and adults. There is no sanitation. In the absence of gutters, waste water runs into the streets and the stream that crosses the settlement. There is no garbage-collection service, so waste is scattered in and around the neighbourhood. Three taps have been installed since 1983. However, they are all located near the entrance to the neighbourhood, making access difficult for many residents.

The organisation of the compound

Although almost all compounds in Samé are based on the principle of a central yard surrounded by living quarters and an outer wall, they are in fact quite varied. Due to the wide diversity in methods of land acquisition, and the long period over which it was settled, the compounds vary greatly in size and shape, with the largest being the oldest.[6] In addition, the way in which space is organised differs from one compound to another. For example, a family who had been living in Samé for almost 30 years had an unusually large yard, with many houses.

In general, buildings are used mostly for sleeping quarters (bedrooms); for entertaining important visitors (chambers); and storing personal items (bedrooms and chambers). Sometimes, an adjoining room is used for storing family belongings. Young children sleep with their parents, and older children generally have a shared bedroom. Rooms tend to be extremely cluttered. Overall, the number of available rooms and their surface area are insufficient for the needs of each family of owners and tenants. Although most activities take place out of doors, almost all women complain that their living quarters are cramped.

All household work takes place out of doors, either in the yard or sometimes outside the compound. When it rains, people stay under the verandah, or in the shed if there is one. The yard is not formally divided among the various residents, and neither is the work carried out in it. The space is used in different ways, depending on the time of day, the activities under way, and the number of people present. The 'right' to use or to appropriate certain spaces for oneself is usually granted by the compound head, but it can vary, depending on the number of people living in the compound and their status. However, this formal division of yard space ends up with women having to deal with the day-to-day details of sharing space for housekeeping work.

Most compound residents who lived with tenants told us that the watchword was tolerance. Space belongs to everybody, and people are expected to accept the implications of this. Everyone knows that it is hard to live with strangers. There are many reasons for dispute. During our interviews, we learned that the main sources of conflict were the use and upkeep of communal infrastructures, such as the kitchen and the toilets, as well as the presence of large numbers of children from different families, and animals.

Decision making and management in the compound

Everyone we interviewed agreed that men choose the site for the family home, and make decisions regarding compound construction and organisation. We found that their criteria for choosing a compound and investing in it do not necessarily coincide with those of the other family members, particularly the women, even though it is they who use the compound most intensively.

The heads of family whom we interviewed (both owners and tenants) claimed that their choices are determined by their ability to pay or their financial interests, their criteria being essentially of an economic nature. For example, the owner of a new compound said that he had not planned for a well, because he could not afford it, his main objective being to house his family. The women of this compound therefore have no choice but to endure the problem of lack of water supply. The owner's mother told us that she was at least happy to see that her son now had his own property, and that he no longer had to pay rent. She knows that she has no power over what decisions are made: 'now my son provides for me, I can no longer make decisions'.

In another case, the family head had been waiting for almost fifteen years to build a wall around his compound. The owner was awaiting the involvement of the urban planning project which was under way in Samé before building: 'Because we're afraid of the urban planning project, that's why we haven't made a wall yet, because the lot allocation takes my compound all up. If I had made a *koko* (wall),[7] they would have torn it down.' The husband was trying to save money by not building the wall. He also probably hoped that the project would, in the end, meet the cost of the wall's construction. In the meantime, the women carry out their daily tasks exposed to the wind, and in full view of passers-by. One of them said: 'I fought with my husband so that he would build the wall. He never agreed to it. He got it into his head that instead of building walls he would build houses, that's what he preferred ... So he had this idea, he said that since he had already been warned that they would tear down a part of the compound, it isn't worthwhile building a wall ... That's why we are

exposed like this, we don't like it, all of the women complained, but ... my husband didn't change his mind.'

In general, it appears that women find themselves living in situations which they have not chosen, and which do not always fulfil their most immediate needs. Nonetheless, even in an environment which an observer might consider hostile, women continue to respect the rules of cleanliness considered necessary to their family's well-being. It is their responsibility to ensure that the family compound is maintained, despite the narrow scope of their decision-making power.

The way in which the organisation and daily maintenance of communal spaces was handled varied from one compound to another. If the owner was living in the compound, he or she usually assumed responsibility for organising life in the buildings and the yard, and his or her standards of hygiene and cleanliness were imposed. In cases where the compound was inhabited only by family members, whether owners or tenants, the head of the household was responsible for the compound. If only tenants lived in the property, they would negotiate together to ensure good maintenance and to avoid confrontations with the owner.

Sharing space among women on a daily basis

The gender-based division of labour determines responsibility for maintaining the compound on a daily basis. Women are expected to ensure the cleanliness of the compound, by taking care of the daily maintenance of the rooms and the yard. As mentioned earlier, on a day-to-day basis the compound space is shared and used mainly by women, and women informally negotiate how communal space is to be shared and maintained. This holds whether their compound is occupied by a single family, or by several families. Meanwhile, men are responsible for constructing and repairing buildings. We met only one man who helped to clean the toilet; he rents out several rooms and is retired, and his wives are elderly. One man told us: '[Whether or not you are in] a rented house or in your own place, women are made only for housework.'

The management of housework within the compound is defined by a system of hierarchical relations between women. The woman head of household generally has the power to organise and oversee the lives of the other compound women, who follow the hierarchy of age and family rank. In the case of extended families, the female head of the family works out the everyday details of housework, and how the personal activities of all the women in the compound can be carried out side by side. In compounds where there are only tenants, women spontaneously arrange how they will live together, without necessarily referring to specific rules. In spite of the fact that women have learned about hygiene in different locations prior to marriage, they generally have similar habits.

The way in which the yard is organised for meal preparation is a good illustration of how the management of space reflects the relationships between those who share the compound. In one huge compound, which was occupied by members of an extended family, three brothers, their wives, their children, and their daughters-in-law, cooking had always been done communally, in and near the only kitchen, which was in the centre of the yard. However, in recent years, the family had had financial difficulties related to the inflation of the cost of living. It was then decided that the family's overall budget would be divided into smaller units, one for each brother, and meals would be taken separately in future.

After this decision was taken, the women of the three units were invited by the men to continue preparing their separate meals in the common kitchen, in order to preserve the appearance of a close-knit family. The male head of the compound explained the situation thus: 'Always with the idea that we are one family, we are brothers, that is why we decided to separate meal preparation, while keeping a single kitchen space [shelter] ... even if there are three meals to prepare.' However, the women of the family chose instead to do their cooking in front of their doors. The words of one of the women in the compound convey the different reasoning of the cooks in the family: 'we cook outdoors because if we went into the kitchen, there would be too many fires ... it would be too smoky, it would be hard to breathe, too uncomfortable, so that's why we prefer to go outside.' It appears that while men focused on the social and cultural importance of retaining an appearance of family unity, the gender division of labour means that the women who actually perform the work of cooking need to negotiate a pragmatic compromise, based on their knowledge of the hazards of cooking in a smoky atmosphere (a hazard documented by Kitts and Hatcher Roberts 1996).

Staying healthy: attitudes and beliefs

Most of the people we interviewed agreed that being healthy is being able to work – that is, to carry out one's usual activities as well as being able to eat well, to rest, to smile, and even to 'joke around' with others. Although most participants defined health in these positive ways, others had different preoccupations, and considered health as an absence of pain, fatigue, or illness.

In addition to these criteria, connected to daily activities, some respondents added that having money is important to maintain good health. While the possession of money is not in itself a factor in health, the lack of worries that comes with having financial resources to fulfil one's responsibilities is.[8] A male informant explained his conception of this relationship: 'A poor person who doesn't have enough money is sick too ... Someone who would like to do things but doesn't have enough money, well, it isn't their body that is lacking, it's money that is, so they are also sick ... When you see what you have to do ... and you can't do it, spiritually you get sick.'

Most people consider getting sick a normal part of life. As an elderly village woman visiting her son in Samé pointed out: 'Humans live in the midst of life and death ... I don't find illness a problem ... often you get sick, often you are healthy. Man is like a tree ... the tree has healthy leaves; when they fall, there can be other leaves. So people get sick often ... or often they're in good health, existence itself justifies it. ... I don't think getting sick is a problem. You have to take care of yourself, even the tree needs water to live and to change its leaves. Man can also get sick. There is illness, good health and then there is death.'

Several ways to stay in good health were also identified. However, even though many ways to avoid illness or to stay healthy were pointed out, many informants believe that God, not humans, is responsible for people's health. One woman told us: 'It is God's will that things are as they are ... even adults, even little children, all get sick one day.' In contrast, others told us that even though, in the end, it is God's will that determines health, human beings also have their share of responsibility: 'Good health isn't just your living environment, you have to take care of yourself to be in good health. God gives us good health, but God also sets limits for us to respect so we don't get sick. So we have to avoid certain conditions so we don't get sick ... that's unavoidable ... there are limits ... God wants us to follow them ... if we don't obey them, we can get sick.'

'Being poor doesn't matter, but you have to be clean'

Respondents felt that the most important factor in staying healthy is cleanliness and, above all, keeping food clean. One woman explained her point of view as follows: 'What you eat, what goes inside of you, has to be clean food, that's important for a person's good health. If you practise it, you can go for a long time without getting sick, cleanliness is very important for good health. Nonetheless, anybody can get sick any time, because it isn't [a human] who decides not to get sick.'

The presence of garbage and waste water in the neighbourhood, including in the brook, was identified as a source of illness during interviews. Several respondents were aware that the presence of polluted water in the neighbourhood encourages the proliferation of flies and mosquitoes, which then contaminate food and bite people, causing a variety of illnesses, such as malaria and diarrhoea. Insects were seen as the main link between garbage and health.

The people surveyed also felt that it was important to keep one's body and clothes clean, both for children and adults, because, as one woman emphasised, 'Dirty clothes on a dirty child can bring a lot of diseases. The human body needs air, if the body is dirty, if the clothes are dirty, it can bring many diseases.'

Our respondents also identified some causes for illness and injuries connected to the everyday environment of the compound and the neighbourhood. For example, since the yard is usually made of earth, or covered in flagstones or rocks, children frequently trip or eat dirt. Moreover, children often get burned when they fall into the fire or on a boiling pot.

Without a doubt, the first rule of health identified by our informants is cleanliness. However, cleanliness is culturally constructed; that is, the way it is defined is based on a number of locally accepted values which do not always coincide with generally accepted norms of hygiene.[9] Moreover, cleanliness does not always reach its objective of maintaining health.

Health practices to ensure family well-being

Urban women's efforts to maintain the family's good health are worth identifying for a better understanding of the role they play in the health of a community. Women's daily practices are a tangible outcome of their understandings of the connection between the quality of their living environment and their family's health. Such daily practices were identified through questions dealing with what it means to be healthy and how one stays in good health. Based on the health 'rules' identified by our informants, we were able to observe how women put them into practice in their daily lives.

'If the water looks dirty, it should be filtered'

There were differing views concerning the drinking water supply and health. Most of our informants said that they drank tap water, and some said illness among children had declined since the installation of taps. Others said they drank well water. One person said she used well water because she found that it tasted better. When asked about the quality of well water, some of our respondents claimed that it was good for drinking. They believe that its quality can be judged simply by its general appearance. When it is a bit coloured, it simply needs to be filtered to rid it of dirt. One man told us: 'If women really think the water is dirty, they bring a good filter [or a white cotton skirt] ... and they filter the water ... You can really see whether or not there are germs in it, you see it on the skirt.' No-one said they drank water from the brook.

Overall, our informants recognised the need to drink clean water, and know how to identify it. However, this basic 'rule' is sometimes difficult to adhere to. For many, it is a question of access, because they live in the western part of Samé, which is fairly far removed from the taps. Collecting water may clash with women's other daily work obligations. For other respondents, it is a question of money: tap water must be paid for, although it is inexpensive (5 CFA francs per pail, and 75 per barrel[10]).

As far as water for household chores, laundry, washing dishes, and bathing is concerned, supply sources are more diverse, because for these purposes water quality is considered less important. Women use water from the source nearest their home, which saves them labour; or a well, a natural spring behind the railway tracks, or the brook. Even though these are activities for which water quality is less crucial, most of our informants agreed that the water from the brook is really dirty, and should not be used. Nevertheless, since the brook is a convenient source of water, some women do use it regularly. In light of our data, it appears that some women tend to put convenience and labour-saving practices before cleanliness. 'Yes, people know what the risks (of disease) are, but they play them down ... because women are faced with problems: you have to wash dishes, you have laundry to do, how are you going to do it? The ground is rocky, there are very few wells in Samé ... so women have to be attracted to the brook. They go there to do dishes or to wash clothes. Here we say: when a woman is close to water, for God's sake, she can't resist bathing.'

People with a relatively high level of education, either a secondary level of schooling or some professional training, tended to be more aware of the issue of water quality, and about questions of hygiene in general. Since men tend, overall, to be better educated than women, yet women are responsible for cleanliness in day-to-day life, this sometimes creates difficulties between the sexes. In several compounds inhabited by government employees, men told us that they had a difficult time insisting that certain basic rules of hygiene be followed, because women do not always listen to their advice. One man even told us that he did not dare to get involved in matters of hygiene, because it is women's domain. As one teacher living in the neighbourhood pointed out, 'The husband has to turn a blind eye, because if he gives orders, it will lead to trouble.' In fact, we observed that women were ostensibly obedient, but in fact made their own decisions when it came to their daily chores. While they had some autonomy within the sphere of their activities, they did not openly question men's orders.

'You can't clean out the inside of your stomach'

It is important to provide one's family with clean food because, as several informants stressed, 'You can't clean out the inside of your stomach.' One man emphasised that the cleanliness of food and water is a woman's responsibility, and therefore depends on the fact that the person who prepares the food is storing and cooking it properly. Women take a variety of precautions to make sure that food is clean (including washing grains and condiments, rinsing utensils, and covering pots and bowls). These careful steps do not, however, always guarantee cleanliness, since most women cook in the open air, at least during most of the year, where food is constantly exposed to wind and dust.

In spite of women's efforts to keep food clean and to respect basic rules of hygiene, there is a risk that children may eat contaminated food. Even though children must wash their hands before eating, they almost always have access to leftovers, and there is no guarantee that their hands are clean. Indeed, since the yards and streets are generally made of earth, it is very difficult to ensure that children are always clean, as one mother explained: ' ... You have to be patient, because every time you clean a child off, if the child needs to get on

the ground to amuse himself, you have to put him [there]. So, he's always dirty, even if you clean him off, he always gets dirty, that's why it takes patience ... Food is the basis for a child's cleanliness; if ... leftovers ... have been left out overnight, and the next day you give them to the child, they can make him sick, give him diarrhoea for instance, and he can get a swollen belly.'

'The mosquitoes are the women'

From observing the Samé area, it might be inferred that residents cannot feel particular responsibility for the cleanliness of collective spaces, since they tend to unload garbage anywhere, as long as it is outside of the compound. It is clear that no one wants to take on the responsibility for the collective management of waste, even though a large portion of the population considers it a nuisance. This collective *laissez-aller*[11] means that it is the women who must find ways to evacuate waste from the compound and who end up being in charge of the problem posed by garbage heaps in the neighbourhood. Day-to-day management of the waste created within the compound is women's business. Since there is no neighbourhood garbage-collection service, and the urban regeneration project has yet to deal with the issue, people dump waste in a variety of places, depending on the location of their house. Speaking of her neighbour's garbage heap, one woman said, 'Since she saw everyone dumping their garbage there, she dumps hers there too.'

Some of our informants did not consider the presence of garbage in the middle of the neighbourhood to be a major problem, since garbage heaps are eventually picked up by farmers for compost. However, other people told us that the garbage smells foul, and encourages the proliferation of insects. Women are identified as culprits for the nuisances associated with piles of garbage. As one Niaréla resident remarked, 'The mosquitoes are the women.' One woman complained that people would dispose of anything on garbage heaps: 'If animals die, people bring them here to dump in the garbage and at night, you can't even sit in your yard to chat because of the stench.'

Men can advise women on where to dispose of garbage, or they can insist that it must not be dumped behind the compound wall, but their decision-making power is, in fact, rather limited, since women generally get rid of garbage when their husbands are not at home, a fact that men told us they are aware of, but in which they prefer not to interfere. It appears that the head of the compound has more influence over tenants than over the women in his own family, since he is able to prohibit certain practices among the former. As far as managing space outside the compound is concerned, men do have the power to intervene if a neighbour dumps his or her garbage near their compound. They would do so by asking the head of the neighbouring household not to do so, and the household head would hand the information down to the women responsible. However, that appears to be the extent of men's power; even if a heap of garbage which comes from several sources develops near their compound, they do not intervene.

Conclusion

Our research clearly highlights the need for taking people's daily domestic practices into account when outlining preventive and curative health programmes. In the case of squatter-settlement restoration projects like the one planned for Samé, making an effort to become acquainted with the residents' motivations can contribute to a better fit between the logic of local people and that of project managers (Geneau and Simard 1995). The actions of Samé residents are informed by logic founded, on the one hand, on their conceptions of health and, on the other hand, on economic motivations or a concern with efficiency. It appears that men and women do not always have the same criteria for organising compounds; men give precedence to economic criteria, while women base their choices on accessibility and labour-saving factors.

Women have the main responsibility for putting the principles of cleanliness and hygiene into practice in the daily maintenance of the compound, although men can make suggestions. In spite of a deeply rooted belief in divine responsibility, women's practices regarding compound organisation and maintenance are intended to ensure the health of family members. Cleanliness constitutes the main rule of health identified in our study. This principle applies to food as well as to the body, and the state of communal spaces. However, the notion of cleanliness did not always coincide with basic rules of hygiene; here as everywhere it is culturally defined, and the practices that ensue from it do not always ensure the family's health in general, or that of children in particular.

In addition to being organised on the basis of gender, responsibilities and decision-making power are shaped by a hierarchy based on whether or not the compound is owner-occupied or leased to tenants. Owners are responsible for constructing and repairing compound buildings, and they make any decisions pertaining to it. Male owners did not always provide the basic conditions requested by women, as in the case of the family whose compound had no walls. Women owners did not have as much opportunity as male owners to make and implement major decisions about their compounds. Among the nine compounds studied in Samé, only two were headed by women; one was a very poor elderly woman who could not afford to repair the buildings, which were in an a state of advanced decay, and the other was the sister of owners living in a neighbouring village. Compounds occupied by tenants were more often neglected than those of owner-occupiers: our study identified many rented buildings in which owners did not make the necessary repairs, or provide basic infrastructures.

Outside the compound, it was evident that Samé residents generally do not feel responsible for the quality of collective spaces in their neighbourhood. The ones who do care are more educated heads of household, and may be either male or female. However, their decisions depend for their implementation on women, who have immediate responsibilities for matters of compound cleanliness and hygiene.

It is generally assumed 'that within the household, there is equal control over resources and decision-making power between the man and the woman in matters affecting the household's livelihood' – but reality is different (Moser 1987). Our conclusions substantiate Moser's point of view. Women, without a doubt, ensure a large part of the daily hygiene and maintenance of the compound, but such responsibilities are not always accompanied by real decision-making power, with the exception of managing day-to-day household activities. Women work and live in an environment which does not always fulfil their immediate needs, and they still have to ensure their family's health.

At the time of the research (1995), Paule Simard was a researcher at the Centre Sahel, Université Laval, Québec, Canada. She is currently working for Abitibi-Témiscamingue Public Health Unit, Direction de la santé publique, RRSSSAT, 1, 9ᵉ Rue Rouyn-Noranda, Québec, Canada, J9X 2A9.
E-mail: paule_simard@ssss.gouv.qc.ca

Maria De Koninck is Professor in the Department of Social and Preventive Medicine, University Laval, Québec, Canada. Département de médecine sociale et préventive, Pavillon de l'Est, Sainte-Foy, Québec Université Laval, Canada, G1K 7P4.
E-mail: maria.dekoninck@msp.ulaval.ca

Notes

1 The study findings presented here were part of a research programme focusing on 'Transcultural conceptions of the environment: the viewpoint of Sahelian women'. Our study was carried out in Samé, the focus of this article, and another poor neighbourhood located in Bamako city centre (Niaréla). The programme was funded by Social Sciences and Humanities Research Council of Canada (project 410-93-1396) and was directed by Maria De Koninck. The research was carried out by Paule Simard, Robert Geneau, and Stéphanie Beauregard (Centre Sahel, Université Laval, Québec, Canada).

2 The research strategy we selected was qualitative, using two main techniques: individual interviews and observation. The advantage of such an approach is that it places social actors at the heart of the definition of their reality. Since we were most interested in women and their practices, using their own words to apprehend their realities proved to be the most effective means of understanding its components (Dagenais 1994). Field work was carried out from January to March, 1995. Each day we observed daily life in both the private and semi-private spaces of the compounds (whether our informants' compounds, or those visited at random), and in collective spaces (streets, riverbanks, market).

3 After a number of fruitless efforts to agree a land-management plan during the 1980s, the *Association communautaire pour le développement de Samé et de Koulininko*, the *Commune III* Mayor's Office, and ALPHALOG, a Malian NGO working in the field of urban planning, arrived at an agreement in 1991 for collaborating on a restoration project. The project objective is to legalise the neighbourhood residents' situation by selling a letter of attribution, confirming

their right to occupy the site (the letter of attribution does not grant property rights: it constitutes a preliminary stage in obtaining a land title which alone grants official ownership to its holder) and to reorganise the neighbourhood in order to make transportation easier and to allow for the construction of basic sanitary structures. A rehousing zone with 280 sites has been planned, first of all to relocate families who have been displaced by new roads and, secondly, to house new residents. The restoration project was studied during the second stage of our research (see Geneau and Simard 1995).

4 All statistics on the city of Bamako have been taken from *Stratégie nationale du logement au Mali. Synthèse* (Berger 1993).

5 It is difficult to evaluate the proportion of owners in relation to tenants, because there are no such statistics available. Our survey and our observations of the neighbourhood suggest that there are more resident owners, and they are most often men. There are, however, many tenants, but they live with the owners. Contrary to the situation downtown, it is exceptional to find compounds in which only tenants live.

6 Since the compound was the basic unit of our study, we chose 15 of them, nine in Samé and six in Niaréla, covering a wide variety of organisational modes. In each compound, the objective was to interview all adults. Overall, 41 people were interviewed (28 women and 13 men).

7 *Koko* is the Bamanan term for the wall surrounding a compound.

8 A Ouagadougou study report specifies the connections between money, which is necessary for purchasing food, and health. Moreover, it is significant that in people's priorities, the theme of health was related to food. In a society in which there is no social safety net, it is understandable that health and food be closely connected. In families with fluctuating budgets, illness inevitably causes an imbalance which can put the whole budget into peril, since most of it is used for subsistence (Gauff Engenieure 1988, 64).

9 A distinction must be made between cleanliness and hygiene, as pointed out by a study carried out in Ouagadougou on conceptions of the causes of diarrhoea (Gauff Engenieure 1988).

10 5 CFA francs = 0.01$US and 75 francs = 0.15 $US.

11 *Laissez-aller* means that every one does whatever he or she wants.

References

Antoine, P., Dubresson, A., and A. Manou-Savina (1987) *Abidjan 'côté cours'*, Paris: Karthala/Orstom.

Beauregard, S. (1996) 'L'impact du phénomène associatif sur les représentations féminines de l'environnement, Bamako (Mali)', Université Laval, Master's thesis.

Berger, J.-L. (1993) *Stratégie nationale du logement au Mali. Synthèse*, Mali: CNUEH-Habitat.

Brundtland, H. (1987) *Our Common Future*, Oxford: Oxford University Press.

Dagenais, H. (1994) 'Méthodologie féministe pour les femmes et le développement', in M.-F. Labrecque (ed.), *L'égalité devant soi, sexes, rapports sociaux et développement international*, Ottawa: IDRC.

Diarra, K. (1992) 'Environnement, conditions de vie et systèmes de santé à Bamako (Mali). Éléments pour une géographie de la santé en milieu urbain', University of Bordeaux-Talence, Ph.D. thesis.

Gauff Ingenieure (1988) *Mesures d'urgence pour l'alimentation en eau potable de la ville de Ouagadougou. Études socio-sanitaires et propositions de mesures*, Burkina Faso: Water Ministry, National Office for Water and Sanitation.

Geneau, R. and P. Simard (1995) *Rapport de recherche présenté à l'association communautaire pour le développement de Samé et de Koulininko et à alphalog.* Québec: Centre Sahel.

Kitts, J. and J. Hatcher Roberts (1996) *The Health Gap*, Ottawa: IDRC.

Monimart, M. (1989) *Femmes du Sahel. La Désertification au Quotidien*, Paris: Karthala/Club Du Sahel.

Momsen, J.H. and V. Kinnaird (eds) (1993) *Different Places, Different Voices. Gender and Development In Africa, Asia And Latin America*, London and New York: Routledge.

Moser, C. (1987) 'Women, human settlements, and housing: a conceptual framework for analysis and policy-making', in C. Moser and L. Peake (eds), *Women, Human Settlements, and Housing*, London and New York: Tavistock Publications.

Schatz, R. and U. Muller (1991) 'Etude sur le prix des travaux d'aménagement destinés aux populations à bas revenus. Exemple de réhabilitation de quartier à Bamako, Samé,' unpublished study.

Simard, P. and G. Diarra (1983) *Discours sur l'environnement et stratégies de développement: points de vue du Nord et du Sud*, Québec: Centre Sahel.

Smith, D.E. (1987) *The Everyday World as Problematic. Feminist Sociology*, Toronto: University Of Toronto Press.

Sontheimer, S. (ed.) (1991) *Women and the Environment: A Reader. Crisis and Development in the Third World*, New York: Monthly Review Press.

Stren, R., *et al.* (1992) *Une problématique urbaine: le défi de l'urbanisation pour l'aide au développement*, Toronto: Centre for Urban and Communities Studies.

Stren, R. and P. McCarney (1992) *Urban Research in the Developing World: Towards an Agenda for the 1990s*, Toronto: Centre for Urban and Communities Studies.

Safe motherhood in the time of AIDS:

the illusion of reproductive 'choice'

Carolyn Baylies

Using data from research in Zambia, and drawing on the broader literature on HIV/AIDS, reproductive health, and gender, this paper examines the difficulties faced by women who wish – or are pressured – to have children, but at the same time want to protect themselves and their children against HIV infection.

'It's frightening to think that I am sitting at home while the "old man" might be wandering, moving from woman to woman to end up bringing HIV/AIDS home to me. I feel that I would even have no children at all so as not to be exposed to the risk of being HIV infected. The only "medicine" is to remain celibate and avoid getting married because that is the most likely situation in which a woman will get infected, considering unfaithful husbands.'

'If I suspected I were HIV-positive, I would stop having children because this would hasten my death. If I suspected my husband was promiscuous I would definitely have no more children with him.'

The comments above reflect women's anxieties about child-bearing when the prevalence of HIV infection is high and suspicions are harboured about partners' sexual behaviour. They were collected in a study carried out in Zambia in 1995, on the impact of AIDS on households in Chipapa, south of Lusaka, and Minga, in the country's Eastern Province.[1]

Given the importance of child-bearing in many societies, and their own desire for children, women often face a stark dilemma. As Marge Berer and Sunanda Ray put it, 'Practising safer sex and trying to get pregnant are not possible at the same time, at least on fertile days, and it may take many months or years for a woman to complete her family' (Berer with Ray 1993, 77). Topouzis and du Guerny comment that, 'If, under certain epidemiological conditions, a woman runs a 25 per cent chance of HIV infection in order to conceive, it follows that if she wants four, five or six children, she runs a very high risk of contracting HIV' (Topouzis and du Guerny 1999, 13). Women repeatedly stare those risks in the face, sometimes preferring not to acknowledge them fully, but often deciding that the costs of forgoing having children are much greater than the potential costs of HIV infection. Both of the women quoted above already had children. Younger, childless women might be less prone to articulate such views so forcibly, or to act on them.

Dilemmas around bearing children are also faced by men, but they have greater immediacy for women, due to the unequal power relations which characterise intimate relationships between men and women. Men tend to have more sexual partners during their lifetime, and more extra-marital encounters. Marriage – and fertility within it – is crucial to many women's economic security. In any given setting, the way such dilemmas are constructed, understood, and worked through is affected by the accessibility of means of protection against infection and/or contraception, opportunities for women's economic autonomy, and the level of HIV prevalence. A woman's age, marital status, level of education, and child-bearing history also have a bearing on the extent to which HIV may jeopardise chances of 'normal' maternity.

Neglect of women during the AIDS epidemic

As the AIDS epidemic gathered momentum in the late 1980s and early 1990s, a number of writers began to speak out about the way women had been neglected by both the medical profession and those involved with HIV prevention. Where they had been taken into account, women tended to be depicted not so much as individuals in their own right, vulnerable to HIV or suffering from illness and needing support, but as responsible for transmitting HIV to innocent children or, in the guise of 'blameworthy' sex workers, to male clients (Patton 1993; Sherr 1993; Carovano 1991). Women continue today to be widely cast in the role of transmitters of the virus. The relative visibility of commercial sex workers has made them a ready target for interventions – and an attractive one, if promoting their safer behaviour allows men to continue to be sexually 'mobile'.

Pregnant women are an even more accessible group for targeting. Throughout the course of the epidemic, the basis for estimates of HIV prevalence in populations has been surveillance testing at ante-natal clinics. The increasing possibility of mother-to-child infections being prevented through medical means has added a compelling logic for pregnant women being tested for HIV on a more routine basis.[2]

Over time, HIV/AIDS prevention campaigns have been directed at women more generally, based on an assumption that women tend to be the guardians of their families' health. But there are limits to such strategies, as women are frequently ill-placed to ensure that prevention messages which call for a reduction in the number of sexual partners, or use of condoms, are put into practice (Hamlin and Reid 1991; Sherr 1996). Only recently has there been a more concerted shift towards targeting men, in recognition of the fact that they 'drive the epidemic' (Foreman 1999). Men are increasingly called on to be responsible (Rivers and Aggleton 1998; Cohen and Reid 1996), via a paternalistic version of moral guardianship of their families' health. In Thailand, for example, male clients have been targeted alongside sex workers, and urged not so much to give up their extra-marital pursuits, as to use condoms, so as to provide some protection not just for themselves (and, incidentally, for sex workers), but also for their wives and children.

However, despite the fact that the position of wives as innocent victims of AIDS has been increasingly highlighted, there is still a large gap between the health and welfare needs of women in the face of AIDS and the attention and protection they actually receive. Their situation can be further complicated, and their ability both to control their fertility and to achieve truly safe motherhood can be jeopardised, when approaches to family planning discourage married women from using condoms as contraception in favour of more effective, hormonal means. On the other hand, in situations in which sexual abstinence and condom-use are designated as the primary means of protection from AIDS, women who wish to have children are frequently left 'with no options at all' (Carovano 1991, 136).

Limits on women's ability to choose

If one considers societal norms about fertility, together with the agendas of family-planning organisations and AIDS-protection campaigns, one can see the dilemmas of women very clearly. The language of choice, preference, planning, and decision-making, often used by health providers, emphasises the reproductive rights that all should enjoy. But these terms often misrepresent what actually occurs. Their use obscures the complexity of a process of negotiating – or failing to negotiate – the nature of sexual activity, which is grounded in power relations, convention, the heat of the moment, and, sometimes, gender violence.

Both men and women may feel aggrieved that they have less control than they might like over fertility 'outcomes', but women typically have far less control than their partners, in spite of terminology which labels many contraceptives 'women-controlled' (Lutalo et al. 2000). Many couples do communicate about having children and about the number of children they would like to have, but as Wolff et al. (2000) demonstrate with reference to a study in Uganda, they often experience difficulty in talking about such issues, use unspoken or indirect cues, or frequently misinterpret their partner's preferences, with men having a greater tendency than women to underestimate their partner's desire to stop having children. Nor, when they discuss such issues, does this necessarily imply equal participation or joint decision making (see also Bauni and Jarabi 2000). It may rather serve as a basis for men to enforce their preferences.

Women typically have even less control over their fertility when accessibility to contraceptives is limited, as is more likely to be the case in rural than urban areas, or where contraceptive use is discouraged by religious dictates. There are considerable differences between countries, reflecting in part the varying scope of national or voluntary-sector family-planning programmes. For example, in 1994, 43 per cent of women aged 20-49 in Zimbabwe reported that they were currently using 'any contraceptive method', while the figure in neighbouring Zambia in 1996 was just 23 per cent (Blanc and Way 1998; Central Statistical Office et al. 1997).

HIV protection within marriage

Across most of Africa and many other parts of the developing world, however, the majority of women do not use 'modern' means of contraception, or indeed any means (Blanc and Way 1998). This amounts to a substantial unmet need for effective fertility control. Many women similarly have limited ability to protect themselves from HIV, not least within marriage, and especially during its early years when families are being built. The power relations which operate in this context are not absolute, and vary from place to place and according to other factors, such as the level of education of partners. But they typically serve to put women at a disadvantage. In the mid-1990s in Zambia, 65 per cent of married women considered themselves to be at risk of getting AIDS, as against 54 per cent of those formerly married and 35 per cent of those never married. Almost all of those married women who considered themselves at moderate or great risk gave as their reason the fact that their husbands had multiple partners. Just under half of all married men also considered themselves at risk of AIDS, but for those who perceived the risk to be moderate or great, the primary reason was, once again, that they had multiple partners (Central Statistical Office *et al.* 1997).

Even when a woman strongly suspects that her partner may be carrying the HIV virus, she may feel that there is little she can do about it. In a focus group in Kenya, one woman despaired, 'There is nothing a woman can do, because it is the man who brought her to that house. She has to submit to her husband for sex. Women don't have any powers to decide on issues concerning sex.' (Bauni and Jarabi 2000) Another woman concurred: 'You will be beaten if you refuse to have sex', while another stated: 'There is nothing I can do because he is my husband, and also, I don't know about what to use.' (Bauni and Jarabi 2000) In the mid-1990s in Zambia, 24 per cent of currently married women said that there was either no way to protect themselves, or that they did not know of any way (Central Statistical Office *et al.* 1997). In the Eastern Province, the figure was 39 per cent. Marital relations may suffer in consequence of anxieties and suspicions around AIDS, and break-ups may occur. However, these seem more typically to involve men sending away wives, than women leaving their husbands (Carpenter *et al.* 1999). The fact that men often re-marry more quickly may account in part for higher rates of HIV among women who have experienced divorce and separation than women who are either single or married (Gregson *et al.* 1997, 1998; Kapiga *et al.* 1998).

When the facilitator in the Zambia research asked women in a focus group in Makungwa, a village, near Minga in the Eastern Province, 'Have you ever heard of a condom?', some said they had, while others demurred. Only one woman said she had ever seen one. The women did not know where or how to get them. But it would matter little, they contended: 'Some, in fact most, men would not agree to use a condom.' And then one asked, 'Are there condoms for women?'

Condoms are a particular issue of contention, as they can be used for both family planning and protection from sexually transmitted infection, but are associated in much of Africa (as elsewhere) with casual encounters or commercial sex. This association has been strengthened by slogans used in AIDS-prevention campaigns in many African settings, which call for abstinence prior to marriage and fidelity within it, and for any lapses through pre-marital or extra-marital encounters to be protected through the use of condoms. In Thailand and India, there have been similarly strong messages promoting the use of condoms outside marriage. The success of such campaigns makes it increasingly difficult for the condom to be promoted as a viable means of protection in sex within marriage. Meanwhile, advocacy of its extra-marital use serves in turn to reinforce the expectation that men (in particular) are liable to stray, and to underline the distinction not so much between what is moral or immoral sex (although that certainly applies in the minds of some), but between reproductive and recreational sex, the former increasingly associated with marriage and the latter with extra-marital encounters. This presumes there to be a difference between men's and women's sexual needs, with men's needs dictating the nature of sexual encounters and the roles which partners assume within them (Holland *et al.* 1998; Giffin 1998).

Women often emphasise their difficulty in persuading their husbands to use condoms (Bauni and Jarabi 2000; Baylies and Bujra 2000), because a request of this nature implies lack of trust. It may be easier to negotiate the use of condoms as a contraceptive, which then offers a secondary benefit of protection from HIV. But once again, the association of condoms with illicit sex can make even this problematic. Both in attempting to secure protection and trying to control fertility, women may resort to secret means. As a woman in Bauni and Jarabi's (2000) study in Kenya commented, such methods were essential, given that husbands only wanted sex and had little interest in family planning. Female condoms would seem to be a possible remedy, since they are 'in the hands of' women. In practice, however, even if they were readily accessible, it is highly unlikely that female condoms could be used without the knowledge of partners; negotiation will still be required. Moreover, in the minds of some, the female condom connotes the same association with 'extra-marital' sex as does the male condom (Kaler 2001). Microbicides which are also spermicides – or which provide protection against infection while permitting pregnancy – may be more promising.

It is not through secretive agency that women are likely to gain genuine control, but rather through challenging and transforming the gender relations which put them at risk in the first place. Without this, and without a change in men's behaviour, the problem of reconciling desired fertility with protection will remain.

Fertility among women who are HIV-positive

Many women do not know whether they or their partners are HIV-positive, and often, with much imprecision, use their children's health as a marker of their own. The anxiety a woman feels may not necessarily impact on her child-bearing, but she may wish to hedge her bets by having fewer children (Baylies 2000; Gregson et al. 1997, 1998) or, as one woman in Minga, Zambia explained, by having them more quickly so that if she becomes ill she will already have completed her family. But what of the situation of those who wish to have children when they already know that they are living with HIV or AIDS?

The situation may have changed substantially for some women elsewhere over recent years. But in Zambia, where few women have access to technical means of conceiving safely or to medication which could prolong lives, there are strong views that HIV-positive women should not have children. As one woman in Chipapa, Zambia, said, 'I would not have any more children if I found that I was positive. What is the point when they will end up dying?' While it overestimates the probability of HIV transmission from a woman to her children, this is a view deeply felt and often repeated, sometimes supplemented with the rationale that the woman's health would deteriorate should she become pregnant and she would also die 'soon'. Such sentiments reflect strong feelings of guilt about children being brought into the world only to face a quick death, and a sensitivity to the costs borne by wider society, even if their lives are short.

Yet even where there is little or no access to new therapies, such is the combination of pressure on women to have children and their own desire to conceive that many women who are aware that they are HIV-positive continue to become pregnant, especially those who are younger or in new relationships (Ryder et al. 2000; Santos et al. 1998). In many cases this is a consequence of a deeply felt need. Reporting on a small study of 21 women in Côte d'Ivoire diagnosed as HIV-positive during pregnancy, Aka-Dago-Akribi et al. (1999) note that even though the women were 'warned' about the possible consequences, their desire for another child remained very strong, except among those who already had at least four. All six who had given birth to only one child wanted another, as did two-thirds of those with two or three children. Only four of the 21 were using condoms. A study of women living with HIV in France found those with African backgrounds more likely to express a desire for more children and to have a child after a positive diagnosis than Caucasian women (Bungener et al. 2000).

A larger study of HIV-positive women in Europe found a higher rate of abortions and lower birth rates among them than within the general population, but a greater chance of pregnancy among those younger and born outside Europe, underlining the extent to which reproductive behaviour is related to cultural and social attitudes (van Benthem *et al.* 2000). [3]

Earlier in the epidemic, Bury (1991, 47) noted that decisions about pregnancy taken by women who are living with HIV are determined by a range of factors other than their own health and that of the child. 'She may wish to have a baby as it may be the only creative thing she has ever done. Knowledge of her HIV status and the realisation that she may die soon may be added reasons for wanting to fulfil herself in some way before she dies, and to leave something of herself after she is gone.' Hepburn (1991, 62) commented along similar lines that while some would prefer not to risk the possibility of a child being infected with HIV, 'Others consider having a child so important that any level of risk would be acceptable', with cultural, moral, or religious factors exerting a strong influence over considerations about contraception or termination.

Women who become pregnant when they are aware of their HIV status may be exercising choice, and, in the relatively rare cases where technical means permit, may be able to do so while their partners remain safe from infection. Where drug therapies are available, they can also minimise the probability of HIV transmission to their children. In many cases, however, factors associated with the context in which women live mean there is no possibility of 'choice' or 'control' over fertility or its outcomes. Fear of abandonment may make women reluctant to inform partners of their HIV status, let alone change their fertility behaviour. In a study in Burkino Faso, for example, this anxiety lay behind the fact that fewer than one-third of women who had been diagnosed with

HIV told their partners about the diagnosis (Issiaka *et al.* 2001; see also Keogh *et al.* 1994; Ryder *et al.* 1991; Aka-Dago-Aribi *et al.* 1999; Santos *et al.* 1998). Marriage or customary unions may be based on affection, but are typically also entered into and sustained for reasons of economic security, which become all the more pressing when women are pregnant, newly delivered, or have a number of young children.

Moreover, some pregnancies among women with HIV may result from pressure from their partners, even when women's partners are informed about their HIV status (Bungener *et al.* 2000). Among the 45 per cent of HIV-positive women studied by Keogh *et al.* (1994) who gave birth over a three-year follow-up period, slightly fewer than half of pregnancies were 'planned', with four of these having been wanted by the male partner only. Lutalo *et al.* (2000) suggest that the couples they studied in Uganda appeared motivated to have children largely in order to meet social obligations, despite risks of transmission, and speculate that this might reflect the patrilineal culture of the area. Although some were using contraception, fewer than half were using condoms. Similar instances of unprotected sex have been found in other studies (Hira *et al.* 1990; Keogh *et al.* 1994; Santos *et al.* 1998) of couples where one or both had been diagnosed with HIV, in some cases as a consequence of their partners' opposition to using protection.

However, this pattern is neither uniform nor universal. While a third of women in Keogh *et al.*'s study were not using condoms, many of the others were. Moreover, there is some evidence of condoms being used for protection, alongside negotiated attempts to conceive in as much safety as possible. Thus, Ryder *et al.* (2000) report on predominantly safe pregnancies among 24 couples (albeit involving one new HIV infection) where women tried to restrict instances of unprotected sex to times when they considered themselves most fertile.

But this was a case involving a high level of support from research and medical teams, which is unavailable to most couples.

Particular problems for young, unmarried women

Particularly complicated dilemmas arise in respect of sexual relations among unmarried young people, not least because this is an area beyond the boundaries of what many regard as 'legitimate fertility' (Garenne et al. 2000). Data from Health and Demographic Surveys conducted during the 1990s indicate that many – in some age groups most – young people in developing countries are not sexually active (Blanc and Way 1998) and a relatively small minority have multiple partners. Moreover, the age of sexual initiation is rising in many societies. However, the gap between age of sexual initiation and age at first marriage is increasing, marking not just the possibility of pregnancy but also the extent of potential danger of HIV infection where sex is unprotected (Blanc and Way 1998). Young women are especially susceptible to HIV infection, in consequence of physiological immaturity, higher susceptibility to other STDs, and vulnerability to non-consensual sex (UNAIDS 1999; Baden and Wach 1998).

Young people are often left in the lurch, targeted by AIDS-prevention campaigns exhorting them to abstain from sex, given incomplete sex education by schools, parents, or traditional educators, and largely excluded from family-planning campaigns (Baylies and Bujra 1999; Garenne et al. 2000). They inhabit a milieu of rapidly changing, contradictory sexual norms with mixed messages from parents, peers, and AIDS campaigners. Significantly, they are often left with limited access to means of either contraception or protection against HIV. Their first sexual encounters are almost always unprotected, and they are more likely than older people to experience contraceptive failure (Blanc and Way 1998).

For young women, choice in respect of both child-bearing and ensuring protection may be particularly problematic. Social pressures may bear heavily upon them, albeit in contradictory ways. Nyanzi et al. (2000) describe how tensions between traditional attitudes towards female chastity and modern notions of sexual freedom complicate the lives of adolescents in Uganda. Gage (1998) notes that, in several African societies, girls are under pressure on the one hand to avoid having children, and on the other to prove their fertility, whether to secure a relationship or to demonstrate themselves to be a desirable partner. Many young people are adopting protective practices, but this is less true of women than men, and, as Baggaley et al. (1997) show in their study of university students in Zambia, it is more likely to occur during casual encounters than with regular partners. Frequently, young people face the future with a high level of fatalism, adopting what appears to their parents to be a brazen attitude, but to their peers a sophisticated realism. They frequently misperceive risks and harbour false confidence about their safety. As Hulton et al. (2000) note in reference to a Uganda study, boys often see sex as natural and predominantly for pleasure and pregnancy as accidental. Adolescent girls may contrive ingenious means of dealing with potential sexual partners, yet show reluctance to introduce condoms into their sexual negotiations, conceding when their partners reject protection on grounds that it hinders male pleasure (Nyanzi et al. 2000).

The possibility of more positive outcomes

The dilemmas facing women who wish to bear children in safety are many and multi-faceted. A few may choose to forego the great satisfaction of having children.

Some will be fortunate enough to secure responsible partners. But most will take risks with their lives, whether after weighing up the odds and deciding that the potential rewards are greater than the probable costs, or preferring to take a more fatalistic stance. However, once women have had one or two children, they may approach the future more cautiously.

There is evidence that some women (and some men) may consider limiting the size of their families, not just in the interests of their own and their partner's safety, but in order to maximise the welfare of their children (Baylies 2000). HIV/AIDS creates uncertainty about parents' ability to survive long enough to ensure their children's welfare. The fewer those children, the greater the chance that they might be reasonably well looked after by relatives. There is also evidence that some women are now choosing to leave husbands suspected of engaging in risky behaviour. In the Zambia research, a young woman in Chipapa, near Lusaka, who was living in her parents' home and looking after her small child, first answered a question about how the threat which HIV posed might affect her child-bearing behaviour by saying she was frightened of getting HIV, and if she felt her spouse was endangering her by being promiscuous, she would not only stop bearing his children, but promptly leave him. But then she elaborated, moving from the hypothetical to the intensely personal: 'In fact, I am divorced, because my ex-husband wanted to have two wives and brought in another woman. I am not interested in a polygamous marriage, and would sooner remain single than risk my life.'

The choice to leave a marriage is bound up with economic considerations, and is influenced by the number and age of the children. In some cases, older children are able to assist their mothers to ensure subsistence, especially in agricultural communities. In other cases, the fewer the children a woman has, the more likely she is to be able to support her family as a lone parent. The mother of a young child in Zambia's Copperbelt explained to a research colleague how she had gone to stay with her mother at the time of the birth. On her return, she discovered that her husband had taken up with a girlfriend, who had been 'taken home for illegally sleeping with him'. He pleaded with his wife for forgiveness, whereupon she demanded that he have an HIV test. When he refused, she left him. 'It is better to be divorced now, when we have only one child, than when we have a lot of children,' she said. Her friend agreed, noting that many women who might otherwise wish to do so 'fail' to leave their husbands because they are concerned about the future of their children (Chabala, field notes, 25 February 1999). The more children they have, the greater their sense that their children's welfare depends on the material security which marriage affords.

In conclusion, sexual practices and identities, which contribute so fundamentally to a sense of cultural stability, often appear to be 'permanent and natural' (Herdt 1997, 8). Yet radical change is possible. HIV presents a challenge to sexual practices and identities, exposing their dangers. There is a certain intransigence in this area, and not a little fatalism; arguments of 'naturalness' and male 'need' prop up structures of inequitable power and privilege. Yet the sexual practices and identities of women and men are continuously undergoing change. The negative and positive potential of this change process is sharply illuminated in the face of AIDS. While young people are placed in particular danger, the greater autonomy they strive for can set the stage for a more considered approach to their future mutual survival. But perhaps the issue can be most forcefully addressed by the generation adjacent to them, and particularly by women who already have at least some children. If their husbands fail to behave 'responsibly', such women may determine that for their own safety and the ultimate welfare of their children, they must go their own way. But they must, in turn, do so responsibly. Of necessity, the HIV/AIDS epidemic forces a sober look at sexual practices and identities, and the power relations which inform them. It has brought some change – although admittedly also some return to older practices. But it will require not just change in behaviour, but much more fundamental change in the nature of gender relations if conceiving children is to be safe for both women and men in future, and for their offspring.

Carolyn Baylies is a Senior Lecturer in Sociology at the University of Leeds, Leeds LS2 9JT, UK.
E-mail: c.l.baylies@leeds.ac.uk

Notes

1 The project involved small surveys, each with 150 participants, focus group discussions, and in-depth interviews with a sub-set of the initial sample. The study was funded under the UK Government's Overseas Development Administration's (now Department for International Development) Links between Population and the Environment Research Programme. Among those involved in the research and its administration deserving particular mention are Veronica Manda, Mbozi Haimbe, Oliver Saasa, Beatrice Liatto-Katundu, Mary Zulu, Epiphano Phiri, Bornwell Maluluka, Edwin Cheelo, and Melanie Ndzinga.

2 While the primary objective of such testing is prevention of paediatric AIDS, in countries where wealth and political will exists, women found to be living with HIV infection may enjoy a secondary, fortuitous benefit via access to anti-retroviral drugs. This is not only the case for women in Europe and North America, but also in countries such as Brazil (see Bergenstrom and Sherr 2000; Santos *et al.* 1998).

3 The studies by Bungener *et al.* (2000) and van Benthem *et al.* (2000) were conducted in the mid-1990s. It is possible that the increased life expectancy that antiretroviral regimes offer will alter HIV-positive women's calculations about having children, offering hope for more 'normal' maternity. But there is insufficient data to know how far this will be the case.

References

Aka-Dago-Akribi, H., Desgrees du Lou, A., Msellati, P., Dossou, R., and C. Welffens-Ekra (1999) 'Issues surrounding reproductive choice for women living with HIV in Abidjan', *Reproductive Health Matters*, 7(13).

Baden, S. and H. Wach (1998) 'Gender, HIV/AIDS transmission, and impacts: a review of issues and evidence', *Bridge*, Report no. 47, Institute of Development Studies, University of Sussex, UK.

Baggaley, R., Drobniewski, F., Pozniak, A., Chipanta, D., Tembo, M., and P. Godfrey-Faussett (1997) 'Knowledge and attitudes to HIV and AIDS and sexual practices among university students in Lusaka, Zambia and London, England: are they so different?', *Journal of the Royal Society of Health*, 117(2): 88-94.

Bauni, E. and B. Jarabi (2000) 'Family planning and sexual behaviour in the era of HIV/AIDS: the case of Nakuru District, Kenya', *Studies in Family Planning* 31(1): 69-80.

Baylies, C. (2000) 'The impact of HIV on family size preference in Zambia', *Reproductive Health Matters*, 8(15)

Baylies, C., Bujra, J., *et al.* (1999) 'Rebels at risk, young women and the shadow of AIDS', in C. Becker, J.-P. Dozon, C. Obbo, and M. Toure (eds), *Experiencing and Understanding AIDS in Africa*, Dakar/Paris: Codesria/Editions Karthala/IRD.

Baylies, C., Bujra, J., and the Gender and AIDS Group (2000) AIDS, *Sexuality and Gender in Africa, Collective Strategies for*

Protection Against AIDS in Tanzania and Zambia, London: Routledge.

Berer, M. with S. Ray (1993) *Women and HIV/AIDS, An International Resource Book*, London: Pandora.

Bergenstrom, A. and L. Sherr (2000) 'A review of HIV testing policies and procedures for pregnant women in public maternity units of Porto Alegre, Rio Grande do Sul, Brazil', *AIDS Care*, 12(2): 177-86.

Blanc, A. and A. Way (1998) 'Sexual behaviour and contraceptive knowledge and use among adolescents in developing countries', *Studies in Family Planning*, 29(2): 106-16.

Bungener, C., Marchand-Gonod, N., and R. Jouvent (2000) 'African and European HIV-positive women: psychological and psychosocial differences', *AIDS Care*, 17(5): 541-8.

Bury, J. (1991) 'Pregnancy, Heterosexual Transmission and Contraception', in Bury, Morrison and McLachlan (eds), *Working With Women and AIDS*, London: Routledge (1992).

Carovano, K. (1991) 'More than mothers and whores: redefining the AIDS prevention needs of women', *International Journal of Health Services*, 21(1): 131-42.

Carpenter, L., Kamali, A., Ruberantwari, A., Malamba, S., and A. Whitworth (1999) 'Rates of HIV-1 transmission within marriage in rural Uganda in relation to the HIV sero-status of the partners', *AIDS*, 13: 1083-9.

Central Statistical Office [Zambia], Ministry of Health, and Macro International, Inc. (1997) *Zambia Demographic and Health Survey 1996*, Calverton MD: Central Statistical Office and Macro International, Inc.

Cohen, D. and E. Reid (1996) 'The Vulnerability of Women: is this a Useful Construct for Policy and Programming?', Issues Paper no. 28, New York: UNDP HIV and Development Programme.

Foreman, M. (ed.) (1999) *AIDS and Men, Taking Risks or Taking Responsibility?* London: Panos/Zed Books.

Gage, A. (1998) 'Sexual activity and contraceptive use: the components of the decision-making process', *Studies in Family Planning*, 29(2): 154-66.

Garenne, M., Tollman, S., and K. Kahn (2000) 'Premarital fertility in rural South Africa: a challenge to existing population policy', *Studies in Family Planning*, 31(1): 47-54.

Giffin, K. (1998) 'Beyond empowerment: heterosexualities and the prevention of AIDS', *Social Science and Medicine*, 46(2): 151-6.

Gregson, S., et al. (1997) 'HIV and fertility change in rural Zimbabwe', *Health Transition Review*, 7(Supp. 2): 89-112.

Gregson, S., et al. (1998). 'Is there evidence for behaviour change in response to AIDS in rural Zimbabwe?', *Social Science and Medicine*, 46(3): 321-30.

Hamlin, J. and E. Reid (1991), 'Women, the HIV Epidemic and Human Rights: a Tragic Imperative', Issues Paper no. 8, New York: UNDP HIV and Development Programme.

Hepburn, M. (1991) 'Pregnancy and HIV, screening, counselling and services', in Judy Bury, Val Morrison, and Sheena McLachlan (eds), *Working with Women with AIDS*, London: Routledge.

Herdt, G. (1997) 'Sexual cultures and population movement: implications for AIDS/STDs', in G. Herdt (ed.), *Sexual Cultures and Migration in the Era of AIDS, Anthropological and Demographic Perspectives*, Oxford: Oxford University Press.

Hira, S., Mangrola, G., Mwale, C., Chintu, C., et al. (1990) 'Apparent vertical transmission of human immunodeficiency virus type 1 by breastfeeding in Zambia', *Journal of Paediatrics*, 117(3): 421-4.

Holland, J., Ramazanoglu, C., Sharpe, S., and R. Thompson (1998) *The Male in the Head, Young People, Heterosexuality and Power*, London: Tufnell Press.

Hulton, L., Cullen, R., and S. Khalokho (2000) 'Perceptions of risk of sexual activity and their consequences among Ugandan adolescents', *Studies in Family Planning*, 31(1): 35-46.

Issiaka, S., Cartoux, M., Ky-Zerbo, O., Tiendrebeogo, S., Meda, N., Daris, F., Van de Perre, P., for the Ditrame Study Group (2001) 'Living with HIV: women's experience in Burkina Faso, West Africa', *AIDS Care*, 13(1): 123-8.

Kaler, A. (2001) '"It's some kind of women's empowerment": the ambiguity of the female condom as a marker of female empowerment', *Social Science and Medicine*, 53(5): 783-96.

Keogh, P., Allen, S., Almedal, C., and B. Temahagili (1994) 'The Social Impact of HIV Infection on Women in Kigali, Rwanda: a Prospective Study', *Social Science and Medicine*, 38(8): 1047-53.

Lutalo, T., Kidugavu, M., Wawer, M., Serwadda, D., Zabin, and R. Gray (2000) 'Trends and determinants of contraceptive use in Rakai District, Uganda 1995-98', *Studies in Family Planning*, 31(3): 217-27.

Nyanzi. S., Pool, R., and J. Kinsman (2000) 'The negotiation of sexual relationships among school pupils in south-western Uganda', *AIDS Care*, 13(1): 83-98.

Patton, C. (1993) '"With champagne and roses": women at risk from/in AIDS discourse', in C. Squire (ed.), *Women and AIDS, Psychological Perspectives*, London: Sage Publications.

Rivers, K. and P. Aggleton (1998) 'Men and the HIV Epidemic', New York: UNDP HIV and Development Programme.

Ryder, R.W., *et al.* (1991) 'Fertility rates in 238 HIV-1-seropositive women in Zaire followed for 3 years post-partum', *AIDS*, 5(12): 1521-7.

Ryder, R., Kamenga, C., Jingu, M., Mbuyi, N., and F. Behets (2000) 'Pregnancy and HIV-1 incidence in 178 married couples with discordant HIV-1 serostatus: additonal experience at an HIV-1 counselling centre in the Democratic Republic of Congo', *Tropical Medicine and International Health*, 5(7): 482-7.

Santos, N., Ventura-Filipe, E., and V. Palva (1998) 'HIV positive women, reproduction and sexuality in Sao Paulo, Brazil', *Reproductive Health Matters*, 6(12)

Sherr, L. (1993) 'HIV testing in pregnancy', in C. Squire (ed.), *Women and AIDS, Psychological Perspectives*, London: Sage Publications.

Sherr, L. (1996) 'Tomorrow's era: gender, psychology and HIV infection', in L. Sherr, C. Hankins, and L. Bennett (eds), *AIDS as a Gender Issue, Psychological Perspectives*, London: Taylor & Francis.

Topouzis, D. and J. du Guerny (1999) 'Sustainable Agricultural/Rural Development and Vulnerability to the AIDS Epidemic', New York: FAO and UNAIDS, UNAIDS Best Practice Collection.

UNAIDS (1999) 'Differences in HIV spread in four sub-Saharan African cities, summary of the multi-site study', *UNAIDS Fact Sheet*, New York: UNAIDS.

van Benthem, B., de Vincenzi, I., Delmas, M.-C., Larsen, C., van den Hoek, A., Prins, M., and the European Study on the Natural History of HIV Infection in Women (2000) 'Pregnancies before and after HIV diagnosis in a European cohort of HIV-infected women', *AIDS*, 14: 2171-8.

Wolff, B., Blanc, A., and J. Ssekamatte-Ssebuliba (2000) 'The role of couple negotiation in unmet need for contraception and the decision to stop childbearing in Uganda', *Studies in Family Planning*, 31(2): 124-37.

Danger and opportunity:
responding to HIV with vision

Kate Butcher and Alice Welbourn

This article presents some examples of successful and innovative community-development work which has focused on HIV and gender relations, and gives a personal view of ways in which the danger of HIV can be used as an opportunity to address many issues which have always been there, but which, until the advent of HIV, few have dared to think about.

Among trainers in participatory approaches to development, there is a legendary indigenous language which uses one character to represent the concepts of both 'danger' and 'opportunity'. This symbol, which simultaneously represents two very different attitudes to a situation, reminds us of different ways in which people have responded to HIV/AIDS. HIV has now been an issue of major concern for at least 20 years and continues to pose immense challenges, which humanity has been unable to meet. Yet many individuals and groups who are infected with HIV, or touched in other ways, have risen to its challenge. One key example is Noerine Kaleeba, who founded TASO in Uganda in 1986 (Hampton 1990). We feel that development workers owe it to extraordinary people like Noerine to consider what opportunities may be presented by the danger of HIV.

The difference between the agendas of health personnel and other development professionals and those groups who are targeted for their attention has been a problematic aspect of much HIV work in the past. Most have set their own agendas in response to HIV, and have developed an 'us and them' approach, focusing mainly on prevention work among groups of people who are viewed as 'vulnerable groups' and from whom workers can distinguish themselves clearly. Sex workers are one such example. However, some programmes and projects have taken a much wider approach, contextualising the health issues inherent in HIV within their social context. Below, we give some examples of such innovative work.

The Working Women's Project: understanding people's own priorities

In Bradford, a city in the north of England, the Working Women's Project was established in early 1991, in response to growing public concerns about HIV. Public funds for the Bradford project were earmarked for 'HIV', and the project was ostensibly conceived to reduce infections within the population of sex workers and beyond. It was widely assumed by the health service and the local authority that in order to stop the spread of HIV infection in the UK population, sex workers (who sometimes refer to themselves as 'working women') should be targeted for HIV education. Of course, as with so many similar projects, it did not take long to establish that sexual health was not a high-priority issue for many of the sex workers. Their priorities were, rather, to avoid arrest by the police and violence from clients, police, and pimps; to care for their families; and to achieve economic solvency. Health was at the bottom of their list. It is unsurprising that sex workers in many other parts of the world share these same priorities.

Responding to the views and agendas of groups 'targeted' for development work necessitates moving beyond a narrow focus on a project, to concentrate on attitudes and approaches. In Bradford, HIV prevention was the agenda of the health authority, and not of the women. As project workers, our job was to navigate the grey waters in between. In Bradford, establishing credibility with the sex workers themselves, and building a project which went some way to meet their needs, involved many years of listening and responding. After the first year, a group of women approached the project staff (of whom Kate Butcher was one) to say that they were heartily sick of reading articles about 'prostitutes', which bore no or little relation to their own experience.

Collectively, it was decided that those women interested would contribute their experiences to a book, which would not be edited in a way which integrated a social analysis, but would rather be a stand-alone book of testimonies 'in our own words', whose contents could therefore neither be refuted or approved: it was simply to be a collection of their own stories in their own words. The book took over two years to produce. It was pulled together from very loosely structured interviews with eleven women. Each chapter begins with a poem written by one of the sex workers, and the final poem is a contribution by a client. The process of putting the book together was an empowering one; women began to see points of commonality in their lives, rather than issues which encouraged competition between them. It was agreed among them that the book should be dedicated to the three women who had died during the first two years of the project, two as a result of violence and one from a drug overdose. It was a powerful reminder of the centrality of violence in sex workers' lives. Those who contributed to the book came together again over a year later, to organise a memorial service for one of their friends who was murdered on the street. Obviously, this was a tragic and traumatic time, but the sex workers were determined to make their voices heard. There is no magic formula to guarantee the success of such an activity, simply the willingness of those employed to work with different communities to listen to people, and to respect them as equals.

The concept of sharing experiences with women was critical to the success of the Working Women's Project. Kate Butcher went on to work in Nepal in a different capacity, but continued her links with sex-work projects. During this time, she ran a workshop with sex workers in Kathmandu for the British Council (Butcher and White 1997). The workshop was designed to help women to identify their major concerns about their work and then to share and develop coping strategies. The common issues of concern to both sets of women were far removed from the HIV-prevention agenda of the professional health staff in their respective countries. As key issues in their lives, the 30 Nepalese sex workers clearly identified violence at work and at home, and intimidation and violence from the police. There was a deep-rooted commonality in the collective experiences of these women from Bradford and Kathmandu. At the end of the week, Kate Butcher invited women to use a hand-held video camera, to send messages to sister sex workers in the UK. They were encouraged to ask questions. They asked about the rates that women charged for their work in Bradford, and recounted their own stories of arrest, or strategies for avoiding violence or police harassment. When I showed the video in Bradford, the women there could scarcely believe the similarity to their own experiences. (They were also amazed that anyone could actually 'do business' in a sari!)

It was only by addressing and recognising the issues fundamental to women's lives that we were subsequently able to go on to work with them on the issues of HIV prevention and improved sexual health. In a sense, we ended up with a reciprocal arrangement between project workers and the women themselves, in which we acknowledged the importance of violence or housing or children in their lives, and they in turn acknowledged the importance of achieving and maintaining a good level of sexual health.

Supporting positive people in their response to HIV

In the past, health and development workers have often viewed people with HIV and those perceived as 'at risk' as objects of blame, or, at best, of pity. Most agencies have assumed that once people are HIV-positive, they are really a lost cause.[1] There are a few notable exceptions who have focused on care and support for those who have HIV, and even fewer who have viewed HIV-positive people, or others in marginalised groups seen as 'at risk', as equal actors who can play a central role in responding positively to the challenge of HIV.

There have been many responses from people living with HIV to negative attitudes towards their condition, including a great frustration with judgemental, insensitive, and irrelevant approaches from health workers. For example, in 1998, the International Community of Women Living with HIV, an NGO founded in 1992,[2] launched its own research project to study the needs and perspectives of positive women, called Voices and Choices (Feldman *et al.*, in press). In Zimbabwe, positive women from many different backgrounds worked together with other women on the steering group, underwent training in interview techniques, and developed their own set of questions for the research project. From work with groups of positive women all over Zimbabwe, key findings included initial reactions of blame and anger from family members; the huge loss of income faced by positive people and their families from loss of property and labour, through both stigma and ill health; lack of access to health care and children's education through poverty and stigma; lack of access to information about *living* with HIV; social expectations which made women powerless to gain access to or use condoms; fears about infecting children; and the impact on widows of male-biased inheritance laws. The women commented that they had gained huge support from other positive women in local peer groups, and that the development of counselling services had also helped them to begin to address some issues concerning unequal gender relations with their husbands. For the most part, however, although HIV-prevention information was widespread, it had never seemed relevant to them before their diagnosis, since they had not seen themselves as being at particular risk of infection.[3] They said information had not given them the tools to address any of the issues with their own partners, either before or since.

Since conducting the Voices and Choices research, many of the HIV-positive women involved have developed the self-confidence to join local health committees, have engaged in public speaking, and have attended workshops on gender violence and other related matters. They have also networked with other relevant groups in Zimbabwe. The experiences of the positive women of Zimbabwe echo the concerns of the sex workers of Nepal and Bradford, raised earlier. They touch on issues of poverty, violence, and stigma; of a wish for children; of lack of choice – a reflection of the huge range of issues relating to gender and poverty which were in existence for many years before the advent of HIV. Now, ironically, HIV is itself becoming such a great threat to health and life that funding is available and there is a preparedness to begin to address these sensitive (often taboo) issues in ways which never before existed.

Nurturing alternative views: involving men in HIV-support services

While gender-related issues affecting women have been a key and growing concern for development and social policy, the resultant programmes and policies have often failed to get to the heart of the problem, which is rooted in intimate relationships between women and men. Transforming the relationships between women and men demands attention to male gender identity, and the role of men in preventing violence and promoting reproductive health. Attention must also be paid to the achievement of other social goals, including responsible parenting. One particular area of taboo for men is the need for them to be engaged in the process of challenging gender-based inequality and gender stereotypes. Men need to be engaged, partly because of their role within families as gatekeepers (if they were not themselves involved and did not agree to the discussions, they could ban their wives from attending discussions about women's

roles – and beat them if they disobeyed), but also because they have their own gender-related concerns and needs in terms of sexual health. Although those working in the field of gender have for many years known and struggled with the need to involve men in gender analysis, and the development of gender-aware policy and practice, there is now an increasing international awareness among (largely male-dominated) senior NGO staff (and large donors too) of the importance of sound gender-based work with men in the fight against HIV. The example below, from Brazil, illustrates how this can be done.

Promundo is an NGO working in the *favelas*[4] of Rio de Janeiro, Brazil (Barker, in press). Its activities include work on gender inequality, health, and issues facing adolescents; prevention of intra-personal violence, including gender-based violence; and provision of support to families living with HIV. Promundo has developed an action-research project to work with young men in a context where domestic violence is widely seen as normal behaviour: a powerful image of manhood for these young men. Women are popularly viewed as sexual objects who must always be faithful, whereas men are entitled to have occasional sexual relationships with other women. Links between domestic and sexual violence are also related to unemployment, a history of physical violence in childhood, and a prevailing silence among men about the violence which they see around them.

When the project was still in its research phase, Promundo staff realised that there were often one or two young men in a discussion group who viewed the world differently, and had the self-confidence to question in front of their peers the established view that violence against women was justifiable in order for men to maintain control over their behaviour. Promundo then developed ways of working with these few young men, helping them to analyse the background of violence in their lives and to explore alternative, more positive ways of behaviour. Some older men, who had already formed a group called 'Male Consciousness', were invited to collaborate in the work, acting as positive role models for the younger men. The latter, in turn, were hired as peer promoters.

The peer promoters and other young men wove their own personal stories into a play and a photo novella, entitled *Cool Your Head Man*. The play, which explores relationships, domestic violence, and health issues, is currently presented widely around the *favelas*, and the photo novella is distributed among the audiences. The photo novella enjoins men to 'reflect before they act, and to cool down when they are angry, rather than use violence'. This project is only in its infancy, but through engaging with these young men, their partners, parents, and opinion leaders, it is beginning to build on those few exceptions to the norm which already existed, to explore different ways of viewing violence in the community. The project is based on the recognition that there is a long way to go to challenge ingrained attitudes to gender relations and violence, but that, through building on existing awareness and through encouraging the development of local materials and performances, a sense of local ownership of the project can be built, which will enable its success to spread.

Working from different starting points: Stepping Stones

Another programme which takes a wider approach to HIV than the narrow health-focused model is Stepping Stones, a training package designed for community-wide use (Welbourn 1995). Initially produced as a resource for rural communities in sub-Saharan Africa, with a strong emphasis on HIV and gender issues, it has now been successfully adapted and translated by various organisations, in many different contexts (Gordon and Phiri 2000).

These local adaptations have been a key part of the success of Stepping Stones. This is because, although the package covers many different issues (such as responses to the use of alcohol; patterns of access to and control of money in the household; gender-based violence; ways of building self-esteem, assertiveness and effective communication skills; and even preparing for death), the central focus of the original manual was HIV. However, as we have tried to show above, HIV is normally not the issue at the front of the minds of the people with whom we may be trying to work. This is true even of people in countries with a high prevalence of HIV, such as Uganda. For instance, after a Stepping Stones workshop there, young women reported that they were now able to negotiate condom use and were glad that they could do so, because it would protect them from ... *pregnancy*. They were more immediately fearful of being expelled from school because of pregnancy than of contracting HIV (personal experience 1996). It follows from this that, if international funders rush in to promote their concerns about HIV (especially in countries where the prevalence – at least officially – is still low), there is a great chance of doing more harm than good.

As an alternative approach, programmes run by the Planned Parenthood Association of South Africa and the South African Medical Research Council Women's Health Unit in South Africa (Jewkes *et al.* 2000), and in Gambia by the Gambian Family Planning Association, the British Medical Research Council, ActionAid, and others, have successfully adapted Stepping Stones to suit local concerns by presenting the package as a fertility-protection programme (Shaw and Jawo 2000). People in both these countries, one with high HIV prevalence, one with still relatively low HIV prevalence, are anxious to maintain their fertility. In Gambia, a polygamous society, there were also fears that Stepping Stones was yet another Western-inspired population-control programme.[5] By presenting Stepping Stones as a programme which will enable couples to have children when they want to do so, as well as protect themselves from the STIs which often cause infertility, staff have successfully developed the package in a manner which has been well received.[6] By starting off with what concerns participants most, facilitators have been able to earn their trust, which has in turn enabled them to go on to address other related issues.

In the programmes of both countries, as elsewhere in contexts in which Stepping Stones has been well adapted and well facilitated, participants have identified the positive outcomes as a reduction in gender violence, increased sharing of household expenditure, an increase in condom use, reduced alcohol consumption, more equitable inheritance, more satisfaction in sexual relations, and a reduced number of sexual partners (Welbourn 1999).[7] The staff in the programmes concerned also comment that it is now possible to find words to talk about issues which until now have been entirely taboo subjects.

It is ironic that, so much money having been spent on population-*reduction* strategies over the past 20 years, an approach to HIV/AIDS prevention which can be presented as a fertility-protection strategy should now show signs of achieving so much. Once more, work on HIV seems to be teaching development and community workers – at last – the importance of beginning with local people's own agendas, rather than with their own.

Supporting traditional service-providers

Another arena where HIV might be beginning to make a difference is the care and support of sick people. Women have long been seen by gender analysts as 'triple providers', in their productive and reproductive roles, and as community-maintenance workers. In caring at home for loved ones who are sick, women yet again bear the brunt of the workload. Pioneering organisations have evolved, offering support to positive people, such as TASO in Uganda (Hampton 1990) and Chikankata in Zambia (Williams 1990). In the mid-1980s, these courageously began to care for people with HIV and AIDS and their families, and provide non-judgemental support services. At that time, their approach was unique. Yet even these organisations, and those which followed their example, have still done little to challenge the traditional gender models which represent women as the sole providers of such support.

However, signs of change are beginning to appear. In Cambodia, for instance, KHANA, the Khmer HIV/AIDS NGO Alliance, is now working with men, not only to raise their awareness of HIV and their role in prevention, but also to promote their role in providing care for the sick. 'Men have a crucial role to play... and the LNGOs are beginning to work with men in their local communities to identify strategies to do so. Peer group discussions raise awareness of issues such as discrimination and human rights and explore the role men can play in meeting care and support needs in the community.' (Sellers *et al.* in press)

The advent of HIV has also raised awareness among development workers of the key role which traditional community healers have to play, both spiritually and physically, in care and support of people with all kinds of problems. While most development workers in the past have kept well clear of traditional healers, believing that their role was to promote a narrow Western biomedical model of health care, some others have begun to work with traditional healers to promote a more holistic approach to HIV. In Uganda in 1992, one innovative group of traditional healers and doctors joined hands to form a new group called THETA (Traditional and

Modern Health Practitioners Together Against AIDS). Displaying mutual respect, trust, and a spirit of openness on both sides, they worked hard to overcome more conventional rivalries and hostilities (Kaleeba *et al.* 2000).

THETA first conducted a study of the efficacy of certain traditional herbs for treating problems common among HIV-positive people, such as herpes zoster and chronic diarrhoea. There were marked improvements in the health of those involved in the study. Subsequently, a second project developed, called THEWA (Traditional Healers, Women and AIDS Prevention), which developed a gender-sensitive, culturally appropriate strategy for educating and counselling people about HIV/AIDS. Out of this then grew a third initiative, which trained healers from eight districts in Uganda as HIV-prevention educators and counsellors. The training sessions, based on the participatory skills in which the trainers themselves had been trained, proved very popular.

An evaluation of THETA in 1997-98 showed some major changes in traditional healers' knowledge of and attitudes towards HIV, their ability to share this knowledge with others, their capacity to counsel others, and their readiness to promote condom use. One spiritualist healer explained: 'We requested our ancestral spirits to understand the serious situation we are in, and they have allowed us to talk about condoms and to promote condoms.' Referrals from traditional healers to Western health-service providers, and *vice versa*, now take place regularly, as each group of providers grows to recognise the limitations of its own services, and the scope of the other's skills. Traditional healers have also supported the development of positive people's own support groups. Above all, they have helped positive people, their families, and communities to cope better with the impact of HIV and to reduce its spread.

Changing attitudes through working with authorities

While providing and facilitating communal, spiritual, and physical support are all crucial elements of a positive response to HIV, the case studies of the Bradford and Nepalese sex workers, and the HIV-positive women in Zimbabwe also reveal their fear of the authorities. The sex workers were concerned about police harassment; the positive women in Zimbabwe were concerned about laws which favour male inheritance systems. Some organisations have adopted strategies to change the attitudes of the authorities, and challenge the discriminatory rules and systems over which they have jurisdiction.

The Musasa Project, a far-sighted and enterprising NGO in Zimbabwe which works to eradicate violence against women, began to work with the police and the judiciary in 1988, with the objective of fostering a greater understanding of the 'rape culture' and tolerance of domestic violence which Musasa argues exists in Zimbabwe (Stewart 1996). Few Zimbabwean women dared to report incidents of violence against them, because women often blamed themselves for these attacks, and the police and members of the judiciary often added to this sense of blame through their insensitive and accusatory responses. Musasa managed to work closely with the police and judiciary to develop new, more private reporting processes which were both quicker and more sensitive to the women's needs. A faster, simpler approach to the whole system was developed with the police, to bring the accused to court, treat what the women said seriously, and prosecute rapists. Musasa highlights the close collaboration with the authorities as a key part of its success. Since those early years, Musasa has developed to do further work with victims of domestic violence.

While Musasa's work did not specifically arise out of an aim to respond to HIV, it now also works closely with organisations such as WASN (discussed earlier), in a collaborative response to HIV. It has begun to focus on the entire range of activities related to HIV and STIs, including counselling and legal services, public education, and advocacy work.[8]

'Mainstreaming' responses to HIV into the work of development agencies

As HIV continues to wreak havoc in the poorest parts of the world, it has taken too long for development workers to recognise that the impact of HIV and AIDS extends far beyond the areas of concern of the formal health sector: the illness and deaths of large parts of the population – including young and middle-aged adults in the prime of their productive years – result in social and economic fragmentation of society. In many ways, the most acute challenges are yet to come, because the time-lag between infection and eventual illness is long, and the enormity of the problem in some parts of the world – for example, South Asia and Eastern Europe – is only now becoming obvious. However, particularly in areas of the world where HIV took root sooner, the social and economic impact of HIV on livelihoods and all other aspects of human life is now evident.

Consequently, many more development workers are now becoming engaged in thinking and planning which integrates HIV-awareness into all aspects of their work. In particular, they are considering ways of communicating the messages about prevention to as many people as possible in as many ways as possible. 'Mainstreaming' HIV offers an opportunity to address a range of issues which seem to fall through the cracks of standard development work: namely how people relate to each other at work and at home, and how destructive situations can be

changed for the good of all. No longer the preserve of formal-sector health workers or health promoters designing their Information, Education, and Communication (IEC) campaigns, HIV-awareness is being mainstreamed into all development activities in a welcome – if tardy – recognition that it is not only people who attend clinics who are vulnerable to HIV, or put others at risk. An opportunity is now opening up to address the issues of intra-personal relationships which have always been a problem, and have always had an impact on people's social and economic well-being, no matter whether there is a high or low prevalence of HIV.

Recently, a training workshop was developed for technical staff and administrators employed by the UK government's Department for International Development (DFID), in an effort to up-date all workers' understanding of HIV and AIDS and to help them to work through the issues which it raises in the workplace (Butcher and Butler 2000). The workshop has been conducted for several departments of DFID in the UK, and also in some of its overseas offices, including those in Nigeria, Pakistan, and India. The package was designed largely to help advisers and technical staff – both British and national – to think more creatively about their work and to identify areas in which they may be able to contribute to the fight against AIDS, whether in the workplace, or through their development programmes in sectors such as health, education, and governance. The workshop provides participants with opportunities to explore the broader implications of HIV, both personally and professionally.

In Pakistan, a country with an apparently low prevalence of HIV, the participants on the workshop course were mostly administrative workers from the UK Foreign Office, working at a local level. They had little responsibility for the development of DFID's programme. Initially, it was felt that the outcomes of the day might be hampered by lack of input from a programme perspective. However, this was not the case. By concentrating in a gender-sensitive and non-threatening environment on what mattered to the participants, other issues were raised which we had overlooked. For instance, one woman mentioned her relief at attending the workshop, which was giving her a better understanding of the epidemic, but also voiced her concern that she would have to talk about HIV with her prospective husband. She wondered how could she do that, in a society where sex is not openly discussed between women and men. Another woman mentioned rape and the concomitant threat of becoming infected. Regarding workplace issues, the two-day session pointed out clearly the responsibility of the employer to provide a confidential and competent counselling service to all employees who may require it. Happily, at the end of the mission two independent external counsellors were identified, and DFID plans to make their skills available to its employees (and their partners, if they wish).

Domestic violence and emotional stress had already been noted as having an impact on work performance, but they had not been addressed in any clear way before. The HIV workshop allowed a frank exchange of ideas and provided an opportunity for participants to discuss these issues. As a result we were able to identify referral points for staff seeking support, whether their concerns were directly connected with HIV or with relationships in general. DFID has now adopted an internal plan to 'continue to raise awareness among staff of HIV/AIDS issues, including their own vulnerability to HIV', and to address care and support issues for staff with HIV (DFID 2001).

Conclusion

It is promising that development organisations, including large international NGOs and major bilateral donors, are now starting to encourage their own staff to make the links between their professional and personal lives, so that at last barriers between 'us and them', which have for so long prevented the acknowledgement of the impact of HIV on the lives of *all* of us, may be removed. There is a danger here that traditional approaches to HIV may be developed as an after-thought to existing projects, such as engineering, water, or forestry projects. The corresponding opportunity is to build on the lessons offered by innovative approaches, like the ones we have described here. Lack of space prevents us from describing many more kinds of intervention – for example, work with religious leaders, with older women on female initiation, with men who have sex with men, or with people in same-sex relationships.

Overall, we have gained from these innovations a greater appreciation of the following needs:

- To involve, whenever possible, the people who are the focus of development and community work, and their loved ones, in the planning and development of needs-based responses. In this article, we have given examples of sex workers, young men, rape survivors, development-agency staff, and HIV-positive people. Whoever they may be, they need to be involved.

- To engage men, as well as women, in the response, in reflection of their traditional roles as gatekeepers, as well as their own sexual and reproductive health needs.

- To develop a gender-aware response which addresses the strategic needs of women and the benefits to both women and men of more equitable access to and control of material goods and services; to engage local people in local production of their own communication materials, in order to ensure a local sense of ownership of the changes they wish to see.

- To develop responses to HIV/AIDS not only in countries where HIV prevalence is already known to be high, but in countries with low prevalence, to keep it that way. This is in recognition of the links between poor sexual health and domestic violence, gender inequalities, and poverty which are already prevalent in many countries.

We have tried to highlight the need for a collaborative, multi-layered response to HIV/AIDS from the development community, from bilateral agencies and civil-society organisations together, both internationally and nationally. This response needs to take place at many levels: at community level, through traditional and formal-sector service provision, through religious and political leadership, through workplace support, and through legal guarantees of the human rights of HIV-positive people and their families. A truly multi-sectoral response is needed, which fully addresses the diversity of causes and consequences of HIV infection. HIV is here now, and there is no more time to lose. By building on the lessons we have already learned we can save time – and lives.

Kate Butcher is currently working as sexual-health adviser to JSI UK. She works closely with DfID as part of the sexual and reproductive health resource centre.
E-mail: kbutcher @jsiuk.com

Alice Welbourn is a writer, trainer, and adviser on gender and participatory approaches to sexual and reproductive health, including HIV.
E-mail: padbourn@aol.com

Notes

1 USAID, for instance, has only recently started to fund care programmes.
2 ICW was established in 1992 by HIV-positive women from 27 countries in response to the lack of support and information available to women diagnosed with HIV infection.
3 This echoes research from India which found that the highest rate of increase in HIV infection was among married monogamous women, who never thought themselves to be at risk of HIV (Gangakhedkar *et al.* 1997).
4 Urban slum areas.
5 AIDS is often known in Africa as 'American Initiative to Discourage Sex'.
6 The Stepping Stones Gambia Adaptation has just been adopted by the government of Gambia as a nationwide community-based initiative.
7 There are local Stepping Stones adaptations and translations in use both in Africa and Asia. See:
http://www.stratshope.org/feedback.html
8 For more recent information about Musasa see, for example:
http://www.qweb.kvinnoforum.se/members/musasa.html

References

Barker, G. (in press) '"Cool your head, man": Results from an action-research initiative to engage young men in preventing gender-based violence in favelas in Rio de Janeiro, Brazil', *Journal of the Society for International Development.*

Butcher, K. and A. Butler (2000) 'Mainstreaming HIV', unpublished paper, John Snow International UK.

Butcher, K. and S. Chapple (1996) *Doing Business*, Bradford Health Authority.

Butcher, K. and K. White (1997) 'Women's empowerment training', *British Council Network Newsletter* no. 14.

DFID(2001) *HIV/AIDS Strategy*. On-line at http://www.dfid.gov.uk

Feldman, R., Manchester, J., and C. Maposhere (in press) 'Positive women: voices and choices' in Cornwall and Welbourn (eds), *Listening to Learn: Participatory Approaches to Sexual and Reproductive Health*, London: Zed Books.

Gangakhedkar, Raman R., Bentley, M.E., Divekar, A.D., *et al.*. (1997) 'Spread of HIV infection in married monogamous women in India', *Journal of the American Medical Association*, 278(23).

Gordon, G. and F. Phiri (2000) 'Moving beyond the "KAP GAP": a community based reproductive health programme in Eastern Province, Zambia', in Cornwall and Welbourn (eds), *From Reproduction to Rights: Participatory Approaches to Sexual and Reproductive Health*, PLA Notes 37, London: IIED.

Hampton, J. (1990) *Living Positively with AIDS: The AIDS Support Organization*, Strategies for Hope no. 2, London: ActionAid.

Jewkes, R., Matubatuba, C., Metsing, D., Ngcobo, E., Makaota, F., Mbhalati, G., Frohlich, J., Wood, K., Kabi, K., Ncube, L., Nduna, N., Jama, N., Moumakoe, P., and S. Raletsemo (2000) *Stepping Stones: Feedback from the Field*. On-line at: http://www.stratshope.org/feedback.html

Kaleeba, N., Kadowe, J. N., Kalinaki, D., and G. Williams (eds) (2000) *Open Secret: People facing up to HIV and AIDS in Uganda*, Strategies for Hope no. 15, London: ActionAid.

Sellers, T., Panhavichetr, P., Chansophal, L., and A. Maclean (in press) 'Promoting the participation of men in community-based HIV/AIDS prevention and care in Cambodia', in Cornwall and Welbourn (eds), *Listening to Learn: Participatory Approaches to Sexual and Reproductive Health*, London: Zed Books.

Shaw, M. and M. Jawo (2000) 'Gambian experiences with Stepping Stones: 1996-99', in Cornwall and Welbourn (eds), *From Reproduction to Rights: Participatory Approaches to Sexual and Reproductive Health*, PLA Notes 37, London: IIED.

Stewart, S. (1996) 'Changing attitudes towards violence against women: the Musasa Project', in Zeidenstein and Moore (eds), *Learning about Sexuality: A Practical Beginning*, New York: Population Council.

Welbourn, A. (1995) *Stepping Stones: A Training Package on HIV, Communication and Relationship Skills*, Strategies for Hope, London: ActionAid.

Welbourn, A. (1999) 'Gender, Sex and HIV: how to address issues that no-one wants to hear about', paper presented at the Geneva Symposium: 'Tant qu'on a la santé', Geneva: DDC, UNESCO, and IUED.

Williams, G. (1990) *From Fear to Hope: AIDS Care and Prevention at Chikankata Hospital, Zambia*, Strategies for Hope no.1, London: ActionAid.

Strengthening grandmother networks to improve community nutrition:

experience from Senegal

**Judi Aubel, Ibrahima Touré, Mamadou Diagne,
Kalala Lazin, El Hadj Alioune Sène, Yirime Faye,
and Mouhamadou Tandia**

In societies in Africa, Asia, Latin America, and the Pacific, older women, or grandmothers, traditionally have considerable influence on maternal and child health at the household level. However, most maternal and child health (MCH) programmes focus exclusively on women of reproductive age. In an MCH project in Senegal, a community study showed that grandmothers and other older women[1] continue to play a leading role in all household MCH decisions and activities. Based on these findings, an innovative, participatory nutrition education strategy was developed, which focused on grandmothers. A follow-up evaluation revealed positive changes in grandmothers' knowledge and advice to younger women, and in the younger women's nutritional practices. The strategy has contributed to the grandmothers' sense of empowerment: it has acknowledged the important role they play in MCH, improved their knowledge and skills, and strengthened their networks of friendship and solidarity with other grandmothers.

In virtually all less-developed countries, community MCH programmes have focused on strengthening the knowledge and practices of women of reproductive age (Santow 1995). However, in all of these societies, the health of women and children is determined not only by women themselves, but also to a great extent by the knowledge, attitudes, roles, and resources of other household members such as older women, fathers, and older siblings. Most MCH programmes do not carefully assess socio-cultural dynamics at the household level (Berman *et al.* 1994), nor do they develop interventions to build on the roles and strategies of other key household and community actors.

Margaret Mead, the famous anthropologist, was one of the first to write about the critical role played by grandparents in transmitting important cultural knowledge from one generation to the next (Mead 1970).

Andreas Fuglesang, a communication theorist, refers to grandmothers as a 'learning institution' in the community (Fuglesang 1982). A study of indigenous learning systems in Senegalese villages concluded that community elders are primary 'learning providers', and that their role is to 'maintain and perpetuate the community's social norms' (Diouf *et al.* 2000, 41). In particular, in households in traditional societies around the world, older women or grandmothers have played – and in most cases continue to play – important roles in MCH. In Africa, a number of studies have documented the influential role of grandmothers in MCH issues in Kenya (Mukuria 1995), Burkina Faso (APAIB/ WINS 1995), Sudan (Aubel *et al.* 1990), the Gambia (Samba and Gittlesohn 1991), Cameroon (Aubel and Ndonko 1989), Niger (Aubel *et al.* 1991), Tunisia (Aubel and Mansour 1989), and

Ghana (Date-Bah 1985). However, in spite of such evidence, MCH policies and programmes in these and other less-developed countries have consistently ignored the role of grandmothers.

At a global level, the fact that most MCH education and nutrition programmes have not involved grandmothers can be explained by the fact that most programmes adopt a narrow focus on promoting individual behaviour change on the part of mothers, and also by negative biases among programme managers regarding the role of grandmothers in household health matters.

Discussions with numerous public health managers and field staff, from developed as well as from less-developed countries, have consistently revealed bias against grandmothers and their role in MCH. It is often argued that in the 21st century, grandmothers no longer influence MCH decision making at the household level. Second, those who admit that grandmothers remain influential often state that their influence is negative rather than positive. This idea is particularly associated with grandmothers' use of traditional remedies, which are assumed to be harmful. The third bias against grandmothers is a view that, because of their age and the fact that most are illiterate, it is impossible for them to learn new things, and to change their practices. Lastly, grandmothers are widely perceived to be dependent recipients of healthcare, rather than experienced resource persons in relation to the health of others. These biases all reflect prejudices against older people. We believe that the combination of these negative stereotypes has significantly contributed to the fact that the experience and potential of grandmothers have not been taken seriously in community health programmes.

The CCF project in Senegal

Since 1998, the Christian Children's Fund (CCF), an international NGO, has been implementing an MCH project in collaboration with the Ministry of Health (MoH) in two districts in the Thiès region of Senegal. When the CCF/MOH team planned the community mobilisation strategy for the project, the influential role of grandmothers in family health matters was discussed, and it was decided to develop a strategy to involve them in MCH activities. This decision was influenced by the findings of a 1996 study on breast-feeding, conducted with the five major ethnic groups in Senegal, in which the first two authors of this article participated. That study concluded that grandmothers play a decisive role in household decision making regarding various maternal and child nutrition practices (MOH/WELLSTART 1996). Although those earlier findings were widely disseminated, no MCH strategies had been developed in Senegal to work directly with grandmothers prior to the CCF initiative discussed here.

Discovering grandmothers' role as MCH protagonists

A preliminary step in the CCF-supported project was to conduct a qualitative community study in order to investigate the role of grandmothers in MCH. In that study, interviews were conducted with young women, grandmothers, men, and community leaders. The study results revealed that grandmothers play a leading role at the family level both in health promotion and illness management. It showed that for all health-related matters they serve as primary advisers to women of reproductive age and their husbands, that they supervise all MCH practices within the family, and that they have considerable responsibility for directly caring for young children on a daily basis. The study findings also showed that family members generally respect grandmothers and have confidence in them due to their age, their vast knowledge and experience, and their genuine commitment to teach and care for the younger generations. Another significant finding was that most grandmothers strongly expressed their interest in learning about the new ideas related to MCH. They insisted that the world was changing and their knowledge was not up-to-date.

Based on the study findings, CCF developed a pilot nutrition education strategy to strengthen the role of the grandmothers in promoting optimal maternal and child nutrition practices within the family and community. More specifically, the objective of the nine month pilot strategy was to encourage grandmothers to integrate a number of new ideas into their repertoire of practices related to maternal and child nutrition.

It is surprising that although numerous earlier studies had been carried out in Senegal on various MCH topics, with the exception of the 1996 breast-feeding study mentioned above, none had clearly revealed the active role played by grandmothers. We believe that the discovery of the grandmothers' role in both the 1996 and CCF studies is due to the unconventional research methodology used, which differs considerably from the approach used in most MCH studies.

Developing an alternative nutrition education strategy

Most nutrition education strategies are based on the concept of individual behaviour change, and on a 'deficits' approach to working with communities. The aim of this approach is to persuade community members to abandon inappropriate traditional nutritional practices and to ignore those who propagate those practices, such as older women (Kretzmann and McKnight 1993).[2] In most cases, directive communication and education methods are used to convey messages to persuade people to adopt prescribed nutritional practices. Such strategies have generally failed to bring about sustained changes in household and community MCH practices. In addition, they have been criticised for being expert-driven and manipulative. In contrast, the grandmother education strategy in Senegal was based on a set of alternative concepts which focus on promoting changes in community norms, on developing community assets and resources, and on the use of participatory learning methods which elicit collective problem solving and critical thinking.

Changing community norms

Research in health education has shown that, 'To have enduring effects, interventions must have an impact on social norms.' (Clark and Mcleroy 1995, 277) Most MCH programmes have ignored these findings, and the fact that in more traditional societies, such as Senegal, individual behaviour is determined to a great extent by group values and norms. The objective of the CCF nutrition education strategy is to promote changes in community norms related to maternal and child nutrition, which will indirectly lead to changes in women's own diet and that of their infants. The strategy works with existing networks of grandmothers, given the collective responsibility that they have for both defining and enforcing community norms related to health and nutrition.

Developing community assets

As mentioned earlier, most nutrition education strategies aim to persuade communities to abandon inappropriate traditional nutritional practices and to ignore those who propagate those practices, such as older women. The grandmother strategy, in contrast, is based on an 'assets' approach, in which the focus is on strengthening the grandmothers' knowledge as an existing community resource. In this case, the emphasis was on grandmother networks (in recognition of the fact that these are already involved in giving advice on nutritional practices) and on community leaders.

Stimulating collective problem solving

The grandmother education strategy was based on the adult education model of learning, in which the process of learning and of change is seen to involve not merely the accumulation of pre-existing information, but the 'construction of knowledge' by the individuals and groups involved (Cranton 1994). Learning is optimised only when people actively and critically analyse both their own experiences, and the alternative solutions proposed to them, which they use to develop their own solutions to real-life problems. This model of learning echoes Freire's beliefs that all meaningful learning must be based on the reality of the learners, and that a problem-posing approach is required to elicit critical thinking. In the grandmother project, group discussion of everyday nutrition-related situations was used to stimulate collective problem solving, and to challenge grandmothers to explore possible strategies to deal with those situations.

The nutrition education strategy

Community sessions with grandmothers

The nutrition education strategy with grandmothers used in Senegal consisted of a series of four group sessions, which were organised with all of the grandmothers and other older women in each village. In addition to the grandmothers, community leaders and community health volunteers drawn from the community also attended these sessions, so that they became informed about the issues discussed, and could provide follow-up support and encouragement to the grandmothers after the sessions. Each of the four sessions dealt with a priority topic related to the nutrition of either women or young children: the workload and diet of pregnant women; breast-feeding; the diet of breast-feeding women; and complementary feeding of young children. A second important component of the strategy involved the follow-up and reinforcement of the nutrition topics discussed in the community sessions, both within families, and at the community level. This follow-up was the responsibility of the community leaders, the community animators, and the leaders of the grandmothers' groups. The leaders of these groups spontaneously emerged during the sessions in each of the villages.

At the outset, when grandmothers were first asked to participate in the nutrition education sessions, many were sceptical. 'We were afraid. We had never before been invited to attend such sessions on the village square.' But when they heard the songs praising them for their role in family health, listened to the stories about their own lives, were asked to share their experiences, and found that their ideas were respected, they gradually felt more and more comfortable. Over time, the grandmothers demonstrated overwhelming interest and enthusiasm for being involved. In most villages, all of the grandmothers attended each of the sessions. At the end of most sessions, they jumped to their feet to dance to the closing songs. This reaction seems to reflect their deep sense of both pleasure and satisfaction with the sessions.

Songs, stories, and discussion

The community sessions with grandmothers involve the use of simple songs, stories, and group discussion; all are familiar and appreciated activities in Senegalese villages.

While these techniques have been used in Senegal and elsewhere in health and nutrition education activities, in this case their use was somewhat different. The content of the songs drew heavily on the findings of the initial community study, regarding grandmothers' practices and role in MCH promotion. Two types of songs had been developed by CCF and MoH staff. First, 'songs of praise' to the grandmothers were developed, to acknowledge the important role they play in family and community health, to show respect for them, and to encourage them to participate in group activities. Each of the community sessions started and ended with the singing of these songs. Here is an example of one of the songs:

In Praise of Grandmother

Dearest Grandmother, dearest Grandmother
You are such a wonderful person, such a
*   wonderful person*
Dearest Grandmother, dearest Grandmother
Your heart is large and compassionate
Dearest Grandmother, dearest Grandmother

The other songs were 'teaching songs', which contain key information on each of the session topics. They were related not only to the ideas promoted by the MoH, but also to beneficial traditional practices. One of the songs appears below:

Grandmother's Advice to a Pregnant Woman

Grandmother, what advice do you give to a
*   pregnant woman?*
I tell her to work less.
Grandmother, what advice do you give to a
*   pregnant woman?*
I tell her to eat more.
Grandmother, what advice do you give to a
*   pregnant woman?*
I tell her to eat beans, peanuts, and green
*   vegetables*

In traditional nutrition education strategies, priority nutritional messages are communicated through a top-down process.[3] In such strategies, the expectation is that community audiences will internalise the messages, which will trigger changes in their behaviour. Stories have sometimes been used as the medium for these top-down messages, telling people how to deal with a given problem. In contrast, in the grandmother activities, problem-posing 'stories without an ending' were used to stimulate discussion on how to end the story and solve the nutrition-related problem. Each story presented a situation in which a nutrition-related problem arises in a community similar to those in which the strategy was carried out.[4]

In line with the findings of the initial community study, in each of the stories the protagonist is a typical grandmother. All of the grandmother characters in the stories are presented as competent and respected women, in keeping with a concept from feminist pedagogy (Belenky *et al.* 1986) that presenting women in a positive light can help overcome certain biases against them. Each of the stories reflects villagers' daily lives, and includes – like the songs – both traditional and new ideas regarding each nutrition topic, for example, breast-feeding.

In order to ensure the systematic discussion and analysis of the story content and to encourage grandmothers to construct their own solutions, a set of open-ended questions was developed for each story. These followed the principles of Kolb's four-stage experiential learning cycle (Kolb 1984). The four stages in Kolb's model of learning are: 1. a concrete experience (in this case, described in the story); 2. observation and reflection on that experience; 3. formulation of conclusions; and 4. discussion of the possibility of putting those conclusions into practice.

Project community animators told the stories and used the prepared questions to guide the discussion and challenge the grandmothers to critically examine the situation presented in the story, and possible solutions. At the end of the sessions, participants were encouraged to continue discussion of the stories with other community members until they reached a consensus on how to solve the problems presented in each story. This turned out to be an excellent mechanism for involving the entire community in discussion of priority maternal and child nutrition issues.

Outcomes of the pilot education strategy

In order to assess the impact of the pilot grandmother education strategy on nutrition knowledge and practices, both quantitative and qualitative data were collected. The two types of data provide complementary information on project outcomes. Quantitative data was collected before and after the educational sessions, through individual interviews with grandmothers on key nutrition knowledge and practices promoted in the sessions.

At the end of the nine month pilot nutrition education strategy, post-test results showed significant increases in grandmothers' knowledge of the recommended nutritional practices. In addition, routine project monitoring data, collected seven months after the grandmother education strategy began, revealed that levels of knowledge and practices of women of reproductive age in villages where the grandmother education activities were carried out were significantly greater than those of women in project-supported villages without these activities. For example, the comparative data from villages with and without the grandmother education strategy showed: women who initiated breast-feeding within the first hour after birth: 79 per cent and 57 per cent respectively; women who were exclusively breast-feeding: 78 per cent and 54 per cent respectively; and women who identified local foods rich in iron: 82 per cent and 64 per cent respectively . This data suggests that grandmothers' acquisition of new knowledge contributed to changes in younger women's knowledge and practices.

Throughout the nine month pilot education strategy, qualitative data was collected through 'process documentation' (Korten 1989)[5] on the participation and feedback from grandmothers and other community actors. At the end of the pilot phase, in-depth interviews were conducted with community leaders, husbands, and younger women, as well as with grandmothers. Analysis of the qualitative information provides insights into the impact which these activities appear to have had, firstly on grandmothers themselves and on community leaders, and secondly on households and on the wider community. Figure 1 summarises these outcomes, which are discussed below.

Impact on grandmothers

Over time, the grandmothers became gradually more open to the new ideas about maternal and child nutrition, and were increasingly willing to re-examine their traditional beliefs and practices and to begin to incorporate the new ideas into their repertoires. Grandmothers' commitment to the new nutritional practices was progressively consolidated as they observed the positive effects of their new advice on pregnant women, new-borns, and infants. According to them, they felt much more confident, or empowered, in their role as health and nutrition advisors within the household and community than before the education strategy activities. A number of grandmother leaders articulated this feeling: 'The grandmother activities have made us feel much stronger than before. Now not only do we have our traditional knowledge and experience, but we also have the knowledge of the doctors.'

The following statement by a traditional birth attendant, who is also a grandmother, describes the dramatic nutrition-related changes that she observed in her village:

Before, when women were pregnant, we made them work extra hard and we told them not to eat too much. We were afraid that if

Figure 1:
Outcomes of participatory nutrition education strategy on community actors and community nutrition norms

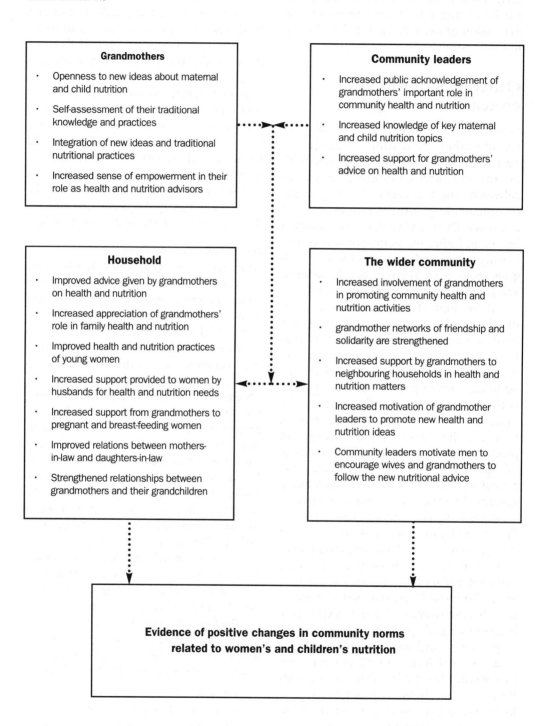

they ate too much, they would gain too much weight, the baby would be too big and that would make the delivery difficult. Since the grandmother activities began, we have learned that many women have difficulty during delivery because they are too weak. Now, all of us are encouraging pregnant women to decrease their workload and to eat more and better than usual. The last women who gave birth in the village didn't have any problems because they were strong. Their babies weighed more at birth and they have been healthier since the birth. Now we put the baby to the breast and give only breast milk for four months. There have been some important changes in our village since the grandmother activities started.

This statement resonates with feedback from individuals in many communities.

Impact on community leaders

In the grandmother strategy, considerable attention was given to involving the formally recognised male community leaders. This is in line with the community development and 'assets' approach adopted in the strategy wherein existing human resources are strengthened. Qualitative evaluation data suggests that this approach affected community leaders in several ways:

- it increased the degree to which they acknowledged that grandmothers have a role in the promotion of maternal and child nutrition;
- it increased their own knowledge of nutritional practices which lead to optimal maternal and child health;
- it increased their support for the advice given by grandmothers at the household and community level.

The following statement by a male community leader shows his satisfaction with the grandmothers' activities, and the role he has assumed in support of the grandmothers:

We make a point of attending all of the grandmother sessions. The sessions are very beneficial, because they allow grandmothers to share ideas between themselves regarding the traditional and new approaches to breast-feeding, women's nutrition etc. This is instructive for us as well. Through these activities their status in the community has increased. We are actively encouraging the grandmothers to participate, to learn, and to try out the new practices.

According to the grandmothers, a major source of motivation for them to participate in the nutrition education activities is the encouragement they receive from the community leaders. Many said that if the leaders did not approve, they would not participate. This feedback supports the need for programmes to adopt an approach in which key influential community actors are involved.

Impact on households

Interviews with younger women, men, and grandmothers themselves, as part of the evaluation of the strategy, indicate that the grandmother strategy has contributed to several outcomes – some quite unexpected – at the household level.

- The strategy appears to have contributed to improving the advice given by grandmothers in keeping with priorities in the nutrition education activities.
- It has increased appreciation on the part of household members of the role played by grandmothers in family health and nutrition.
- It has improved health and nutrition practices among young women, and increased support from husbands for family health and nutrition needs.
- It has increased moral and material support from grandmothers to pregnant and breast-feeding women.
- It has improved relationships between mothers-in-law and daughters-in-law, and has strengthened relationships between grandmothers and their grandchildren.

In all villages, the feedback from both younger women and their husbands regarding the grandmother nutrition education strategy was very positive. In the final group interviews, virtually all of the younger women reported dramatic changes in grandmothers' attitudes, advice, and practices. They said that these changes have not only contributed to visible improvements in their own health, but have also made their lives much easier.

Now, the advice the grandmothers give us includes both traditional and modern ideas. Now, when you are pregnant, they tell you to eat more and to work less. Before, there were certain foods they told us not to eat, and they forbade us from snacking between meals. Now, they tell us to eat more and especially green leafy vegetables, beans, and small dried fish so that we'll be strong when we deliver our babies. Before, each woman had to do her own work. Now, when a woman is pregnant they ask other women in the family to help out, or they take on more of your work themselves. Now they understand us better, and that's why we feel closer to them.
(Woman with a two-month old baby)

Impact on the wider community

The qualitative evaluation data also indicated that the grandmother education strategy has had an impact on various community actors, and the relationships between them. In the villages where the nutrition education activities have been carried out, grandmothers have become increasingly involved both in encouraging younger women to participate in health and nutrition promotion activities such as growth monitoring, vaccinations, and cooking demonstrations, and in participating in these activities themselves. According to the grandmothers, the strategy has strengthened their sense of friendship and solidarity within their peer network, and has also encouraged them to be more supportive of neighbouring households as regards health and nutrition matters.

During the educational sessions, in all villages, the grandmother leaders were the first among the grandmothers to propose adoption of the new ideas on nutrition, and they have become increasingly active in promoting the new ideas among other grandmothers and older women. Lastly, many of the community leaders are motivating men to encourage their wives and mothers or grandmothers to follow the new nutritional advice. One of the community leaders proudly told a story about how one of the grandmothers from his village was actively involved in promoting the new ideas she learned in the grandmother sessions in a neighbouring village.

To sum up, the evaluation data provide convincing evidence of positive outcomes of the nutrition education strategy at several levels. The multi-level outcomes seem to have to contributed to changes observed in community nutrition norms related to the four priority nutrition topics addressed in the strategy. Based on the very positive results of the pilot grandmother nutrition education strategy, CCF is now extending it to all of the villages supported by the project.

Conclusions

In the innovative nutrition education strategy reported here, grandmother networks were the focus of participatory learning activities that aimed to promote changes in community nutrition norms and, indirectly, to promote changes in younger women's nutritional practices. The evaluation of the nine month pilot strategy showed significant increases in grandmothers' knowledge of the priority nutrition concepts, dramatic changes in the advice they give to pregnant and breast-feeding women, and observable changes in younger women's nutritional practices based on the grandmothers' updated advice.

The nutrition education strategy incorporates several approaches that have been identified as contributing to sustainable health and nutrition promotion efforts, namely strengthening existing community actors and structures, promoting changes in community norms, and using low-cost, culturally adapted approaches. We believe that the impressive, and perhaps unprecedented, results of this innovative nutrition education project can be attributed in the main to two major factors: the unconventional educational methodology, and the development of previously untapped community resources. The non-formal education methodology, using songs, open-ended stories, and group discussion, required grandmothers to examine critically their traditional practices, exposed them to new ideas, and encouraged them to consider the possibility of integrating the two. Through this process, the grandmothers not only gained new knowledge and developed their own strategies for dealing with community nutrition problems, but also acquired a sense of empowerment, as members of networks of health and nutrition advisers recognised by the community.

The second major facet that appears to explain the positive impact of the strategy is the fact that influential, but previously untapped, community resources, namely grandmothers and community leaders, were strengthened in their role in health promotion through the process. Through the nutrition education activities, the role of grandmothers in health and nutrition promotion was publicly recognised, and they received strong support from community leaders. The intrinsic commitment of the grandmothers to the wellbeing of women and children in the community was reinforced. The efforts to acknowledge and strengthen these important women met with broad and enthusiastic approval from the wider community, which contributed to the positive outcomes both within and beyond the household level.

We believe that in many other cultural contexts, efforts to strengthen the role of grandmothers in MCH would release this untapped potential, which could have a significant and sustainable impact on maternal and child health norms and practices. In an earlier health education project in Laos, use of the same informal education methodology with grandmothers led to similar outcomes in terms of grandmothers' learning and empowerment (Aubel and Sihalathavong 2001).

In conclusion, we consider that the greatest obstacle to improving the contribution of grandmothers to MCH does not come from grandmothers themselves, but rather from international and national health organisations that continue to ignore the potential of these experienced and committed health promoters. While grandmothers and older women themselves have demonstrated their openness to such collaborative ventures, are policy-makers and funders able to step out of their traditional paradigm and take the grandmothers seriously?

Judi Aubel, PhD, MPH, is an independent consultant in participatory approaches to qualitative research, health education, training, and evaluation. She has worked in community health programmes, primarily with NGOs in West Africa, but also in Latin America, Asia, and the Pacific.
E-mail: jatao@is.com.fj or judiaubel@hotmail.com

All other authors are CCF project staff. Ibrahima Touré is Training and Social Mobilisation Co-ordinator; Mamadou Diagne is Project Director; Kalala Lazin is Evaluation Co-ordinator; and El Hadj Alioune Sène, Yirime Faye, and Mouhamadou Tandia are community animators.
E-mail: ccfcanah@telecomplus.sn

Notes

1 The term 'grandmother' is used to refer not only to biological grandmothers, but also to other experienced women who serve as advisers to younger women on various household issues.

2 Kretzmann and McKnight (1993) point out the difference between a problem-based or 'deficits' approach to working with communities and an 'assets' approach. In the latter approach the focus is on identifying and reinforcing community strengths and resources which include leaders, groups, and individuals with special skills.

3 Freire called this a 'banking' approach to teaching in which the teacher instructs students on what to do. He contrasted this with a 'problem-posing' approach in which 'learners' are expected to formulate their own solutions (Freire 1970).

4 This is in keeping with Freire's use of teaching 'codes' (Freire 1970) and Brookfield's use of 'critical incidents' (Brookfield 1991).

5 'Process documentation' is a qualitative data collection technique which involves taking notes on an ongoing basis to describe the implementation of a strategy or project. It can include statements made by participants, descriptions of interactions between people and observations. (Korten 1989)

References

APAIB/WINS (1995) *Santé et nutrition des mères et des enfants dans la Province de Bazega*, Ouagadougou, Burkina Faso: WINS.

Aubel, J., Alzouma, E.H.M., Djabel, I., Ibrahim, S., and B. Coulibaly (1991) 'From qualitative community data collection to program design: health education planning in Niger', *International Quarterly of Community Health Education*, 11(40):345-69.

Aubel, J. and D. Sihalathavong (2001) 'Participatory communication to strengthen the role of grandmothers in child health: an alternative paradigm for health education and health communication', in press, *Journal of International Communication*.

Aubel, J. and M. Mansour (1989) 'Qualitative community health research: a Tunisian example', *Health Policy & Planning*, 4:244-56.

Aubel, J. and F. Ndonko (1989) *Etude sur les maladies diarrhéiques auprès du personnel de santé*, PNLMD, Yaoundé, Cameroon: Ministère de la Santé.

Aubel J., Rabei, H., and M. Mukhtar (1990) 'Report of Qualitative Community Study on Diarrhoeal Disease', Khartoum: MoH/UNICEF.

Belenky, M. F., Clinchy, B.M., Rape-Goldberger, N., and J. M. Tarule (1986) *Women's Ways of Knowing: The Development of Self, Voice and Mind*, New York: Basic Books.

Berman, P., Kendall, C., and K. Bhattacharyya (1994) 'The household production of health: integrating social science perspectives on micro-level health determinants', *Social Science and Medicine*, 38(2):205-15.

Brookfield, S.D. (1991) *Developing Critical Thinkers: Challenging Adults to Explore Alternative Ways of Thinking and Acting*, San Francisco: Jossey-Bass.

Chrisman, N.J. (1977) 'The health seeking process: an approach to the natural history of illness', *Culture, Medicine and Psychiatry*, 1:351-77.

Clark, N.M. and K.R. Mcleroy (1995) 'Creating capacity through health education: what we know and what we don't', *Health Education Quarterly*, 22(3): 273-89.

Cranton, P. (1994) *Understanding and Promoting Transformative Learning: A Guide for Educators of Adults*, San Francisco: Jossey-Bass.

Date-Bah, E. (1985) 'Sex segregation and discrimination in Accra-Tema: causes and consequences', in R. Anker. and C. Hein, *Sex Inequalities in Urban Employment in the Third World*, New York: St. Martin's Press.

Diouf, W., Sheckley, B.G., and M. Kehrhahn (2000) 'Adult learning in a non-western context: the influence of culture in a Senegalese farming village', *Adult Education Quarterly*, 51(1):32-44.

Freire, P. (1970) *Pedagogy of the Oppressed*, New York: Continuum.

Fuglesang, A. (1982), *About Understanding: Ideas and Observations on Cross-cultural Understanding*, Uppsala: Dag Hammarskjöld Foundation.

Kolb, D.A. (1984) *Experiential Learning: Experience as a Source of Learning and Development*, Englewood Cliffs, New Jersey: Prentice-Hall, Inc.

Korten, D.C. (1989) 'Social science in the service of social transformation', in C.C. Veneracion (ed.), *A Decade of Process Documentation Research: Reflections and Synthesis*, Manila: Institute of Philippine Culture, Ateneo de Manila University.

Kretzmann, J.P. and J.L. McKnight (1993) *Building Communities from the Inside Out: A Path Toward Finding and Mobilizing a Community's Assets*, Evanston: Asset-Based Community Development Institute/Institute for Policy Research, Northwestern University.

Mead, M. (1970) *Culture & Commitment: A Study of the Generation Gap*, New York: Natural History Press, Doubleday & Co..

Mcleroy K.R., Bibeau, D., Steckler, A., and K. Glanz (1988) 'An ecological perspective on health promotion programs', *Health Education Quarterly*, 15(4): 351-77.

MOH/WELLSTART (1996) *La femme, son travail et l'alimentation du jeune enfant*, Dakar, Senegal: Ministère de la Santé.

Mukuria, A.G. (1999) *Exclusive Breastfeeding and the Role of Social Support and Social Networks in a Low Income Urban Community in Nairobi, Kenya*, PhD dissertation, Baltimore: Johns Hopkins University, School of Hygiene and Public Health.

Samba, K. and J. Gittlesohn (1991) *Improving Child Feeding Practices in The Gambia*, GAFNA SDC Technical Note no.1, Banjul: GAFNA.

Santow, G. (1995) 'Social roles and physical health: the case of female disadvantage in poor countries', *Social Science and Medicine*, 40(2):147-61.

Teaching about gender, health, and communicable disease:

experiences and challenges

Rachel Tolhurst and Sally Theobald

This article looks at the challenges and opportunities we have encountered while teaching a short course on gender, health, and communicable disease. The course is aimed at health policy-makers, planners, and managers from national ministries, international and national health organisations, and non-governmental organisations (NGOs). It ran for the first time in April 2000, with participants from Asia, Africa, and Europe. In this article, we explore some of the gender issues that arise in working to prevent and treat communicable disease, and discuss the process, materials, and concepts used in the course.

In recent years, there has been a growing understanding of how people's gender identity determines the nature of their ill-health, vulnerability to disease, their ability to prevent disease, and their access to health care. This focus on the gendered aspects of communicable disease has come about partly through increasing research and analysis on HIV/AIDS during the past decade, which has revealed striking differences in women's and men's experience of the disease. Researchers have now begun to direct their focus at exploring the extent to which gender shapes the experience of other infectious diseases. The short course in 'Gender, Health, and Communicable Disease' at the Liverpool School of Tropical Medicine, UK, was conceived in 1999. The course is run by the Gender and Health Group,[1] and was developed in response to a perceived lack of awareness on the part of development policy-makers and planners of the links between gender issues and communicable disease. It has a specific focus on gender

issues in infectious diseases, such as TB, malaria, and sexually transmitted diseases (STDs), and on the implications of a gender analysis for health systems[2] development.

Gender identities, roles, and relations shape women's and men's vulnerability to illness. For example, a malaria prevention scheme in Benin which promoted the use of bed-nets, conducted research into non-use of nets. Lack of access to cash as a factor in the non-use of nets was mentioned by women, but not by men. The research study found that women are less likely than men to have control over household income (Rashed *et al.* 1999). In the case of HIV/AIDS, the interaction between social and biological vulnerabilities leads to gender differences in the risk of infection with HIV (Zierler and Krieger 1997). Biologically, women (in particular, young women) are at greater risk of infection through heterosexual intercourse. Gender identities, norms, roles, and relations influence both women's and men's vulnerability to HIV and other STDs in different ways by shaping the negotiation of sexual relationships and practices. Men and women of different ages therefore have differing sources and levels of risk of infection. In rural KwaZulu Natal, South Africa, in 1992, a community-based cross-sectional seroprevalence survey found that rates of infection were higher amongst girls and women until the 20-24 age group, while they were higher for men in the 25-29 year group and above (Karim and Karim 1999).

Gender concerns also influence how individuals, households, and communities respond to ill-health. Worldwide each year, between 1.5 and 2.1 men to every one woman is diagnosed with TB (Dolin 1998). This statistical imbalance may be, in part, due to the way in which gender roles affect vulnerability to TB, but it is also due to the fact that women face more barriers to accessing diagnosis and health care. Diagnosis requires repeated visits to a health facility with appropriate equipment and expertise (often a district hospital), and treatment requires drug therapy for a minimum of six months, which should be observed by a health worker or trained volunteer, usually requiring visits to the nearest trained provider. The accessibility of this for an individual will depend on factors such as their financial resources, access to transport, social mobility, their ability to take time off work and the opportunity costs of doing so, the importance of good health for the continuation of work, and their decision-making power within the household. All of these considerations have a gender dimension. Recent research has found that the proportion of female TB cases identified rises significantly when TB cases are actively sought out in the community, instead of only reporting cases where individuals have sought health care and subsequently been diagnosed with TB (Dolin 1998).

Gender roles affect the burden of ill-health for women and men. In KwaZulu Natal, where the HIV prevalence rate has been found to be 26.9 per cent, there is an increasing emphasis on home-based care due to the excessive strain placed on health facilities. This means that women are taking on the majority of the heavier burden of care in the household, which has implications for their own health, welfare, and workloads that are not always considered by planners (Kempkes 1999).

Part 1: Introduction to gender and health

On the first morning of the course, we ask the participants about their hopes and fears about the course, and go on to brainstorm about the ground rules that we expect everyone to follow throughout the course. Gender training typically includes a lot of group work, and reflection on both personal and professional experiences. Participants' own gender identities and values can be a source of conflict in later discussions,[3] so setting ground rules at the outset is an obvious strategy to ensure that the course is a 'safe space'.

Analysing case studies

One of the first tasks of the course is to begin to identify some of the ways in which gender issues can interact with communicable disease. These interactions are varied, complex, and can vary significantly in different settings. Personal stories can be a powerful way for participants to relate to, and reflect on, individual experiences of the gendered nature of communicable disease. We use vignettes showing how different communicable diseases affect the lives of women, men, girls, and boys in a variety of geographical contexts. An example telling the story of one woman, Nora, is included here:

By this stage, I knew Gerry often 'met with' girlfriends at beer halls and hotels. He was a ladies' man. I didn't like it, but it was inevitable, and I knew if I mentioned it to him he would become angry. My friend,

Mary, told me I should suggest using condoms. If I did that he would accuse me of infidelity, or charge me with accusing him of infidelity. If I asked him to use condoms with his girlfriends, that would reveal I knew about them. Again, that would make him angry. I needed Gerry to support the children with money for food and clothes, and I decided to talk to him about HIV in a general way. He dismissed what I was saying and told me HIV didn't exist in our area.

When Tinashe was three years old, I became ill. By that time, Gerry didn't love me any more. He said I was using all his money – staying in hospital and not looking after the kids at home. His sister came and said I was 'culturally infected', and should be sent back to my parents. Gerry said he couldn't keep me any more, so for months I was on my own, looking after the children and selling tomatoes and fruit to raise money for the bus fare back to my parents' home. My mother looked after me, but no one knew what was wrong. I was ill for six months, but I recovered and returned to Harare. By this time, Gerry started getting ill. He went for tests which showed he was HIV-positive, but he never told me. One day I told it to him straight. We were just talking and I asked him, 'Do you remember when I got ill and you told me to go back to my parents? You never took care of me, my dear, so now you are the one who is ill, [and] you must go to your parents.' I tried to chase him away. He refused and said, 'Men can't keep wives while they are sick, but you can keep men.'

Nora's story brings out a range of gender issues in HIV transmission and responses to HIV/AIDS. These include expectations and acceptance of infidelity, difficulties of discussing condom use, especially in the context of women's socio-economic dependency on men, gender norms about caring, and double standards in the responses of families and partners to women with HIV/AIDS.

During the presentation of a case study, and subsequent analysis by the participants, we need to avoid suggesting that all these experiences happen to all women or men in all contexts, while simultaneously pulling out general themes. One way of doing this is to ask participants how women's and men's experiences and reactions to the scenario presented in the case study may be similar or different in the cultural backgrounds (for example, country, class, ethnicity, or location) with which they are familiar. This can provoke a discussion about the ways in which gender roles and relations are constructed and experienced in different groups. Gender analysis should be a personal as well as a conceptual endeavour, and choosing materials that participants can relate to is one way in which to encourage discussions which draw on participants' own experiences and ideas.

Another challenge is to find varied materials. We found it relatively easy to obtain case studies discussing African women's experiences of and responses to STDs (as in Nora's story), but little from a personal perspective that focused on men and STDs, or on women's or men's experiences of other communicable diseases such as TB or malaria. Some of the likely reasons for the predominance of materials on HIV are as follows:

- An analysis of the HIV/AIDS epidemic necessarily involves the analysis of inter-personal relationships, because HIV is predominantly sexually transmitted.

- Women's groups from both the North and South have campaigned about the impact of HIV on women. The clear social implications of the disease have encouraged involvement from civil society, and the development of inter-sectoral approaches, in contrast to the dominance of scientists in the study and control of malaria and TB.

- The dramatic nature of HIV/AIDS in terms of morbidity and mortality, and its potential to affect those in the North as well as in the South, have probably facilitated the concentration of global concern and resources (largely northern) on understanding and combating it.

In line with the above, we have found that throughout the course, the majority of students have been more interested in focusing on HIV/AIDS than on other communicable diseases. To develop alternative material that will stimulate interest in other diseases, we are currently collaborating with the Institute of Population and Social Research, Mahidol University, Bangkok, to develop case study teaching material focusing on women's and men's experiences of TB in Kanchanaburi Province, Thailand.

Another challenge for the course facilitators is to show that gender issues affect men's health and health care, as well as women's. The challenge is to encourage participants to apply gender analysis to both women's and men's health, without implying that there are no imbalances in power relations between women and men. We do not want to move away from a feminist analysis to an implication that women's and men's situations and experiences are 'equal but different'. Since all participants cannot be assumed to be in sympathy with feminist principles, there is a temptation to present the case for female disadvantage in order to ensure that we retain a focus on the goal of gender equity. However, a more sophisticated analysis also accepts the importance of analysing the relationship between masculinity and health, and the existence of male disadvantage in relation to health in particular contexts and in relation to particular issues. This is an ongoing dilemma, which is not limited to our analysis of vignettes.

Problem trees

We use problem trees to encourage participants to identify and analyse gender and health issues in their own situations. These are useful tools for exploring specific health problems, and the relationship between cause and effect. They can be constructed by individuals, and can also be used by teams, and as a tool for participatory analysis with groups of people who experience the problem under discussion.

Each individual participant creates a 'tree' for a problem that concerns her or him. Participants can use this tree to analyse specific health problems, systems-related problems (such as lack of gender awareness among health staff), or problems of interaction between community and health systems (such as low utilisation of services). Problems may be specifically related to gender differences (for example, in reported TB cases), or they may have contributing factors related to gender-based inequality (such as child mortality due to malaria, where women have responsibility for accessing health care for their children but often lack adequate control over resources to be able to do this promptly). Figure 1 shows a problem tree addressing the high prevalence rate of HIV among young women aged 15-19, as opposed to their male peers. The problem tree is a useful tool for stimulating thought and discussion about the nature of problems facing participants in their working situations. For example, one participant commented: 'The use of a problem tree as a research and planning tool was very effective as it linked causes of a disease/problem to the effects. This will help in prioritising areas of focus in planning and interventions.' (Course evaluation 2000)

We have found that gender sensitivity and specificity can be all too easily lost in problem tree analyses, however. It is possible to maintain a gender perspective on the issue if the problem analysed relates specifically to gender or if it is framed in a gender-specific way (as in the example included), but this 'gender lens' tends to

Figure 1
HIV among women in Malawi: problem tree
Mette Ostergaard Strandlod

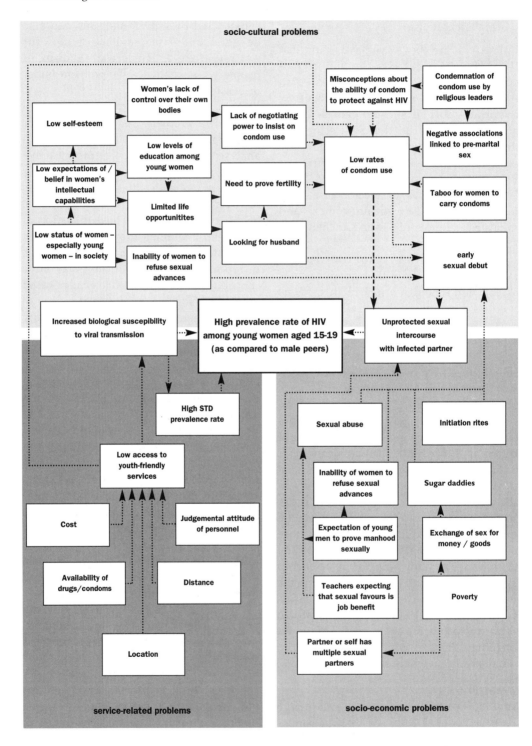

be lost where the problem was framed in a general way, even where gender inequalities are clearly integral to the issue (for example, low use of family planning).

On reflection, the problem tree seems only to be useful in building a gender analysis at this stage of the course if the participants have already been able to reflect on some of the gender issues involved. This suggests to us that participants need more space for sharing ideas drawn from their own work and lives about ways in which gender affects women's and men's experiences of, and responses to, health issues. This has implications, too, for using the tool in the different contexts of programme planning or policy-making, where the facilitator would need to have an in-depth understanding of gender issues in relation to the problem at hand. Perhaps the problem tree is best used after a general introduction to gender issues.

Thematic group assignments

The next step in the course is to introduce the participants to some ways of analysing the relationship between gender relations, gender-based inequality, and specific diseases. Groups of participants are given selected readings from a range of different sources on TB, HIV/AIDS, and malaria, and asked to present an overview of the theory and knowledge about gender issues in relation to each disease. Readings selected include international literature reviews and country specific studies, and are based on both qualitative and quantitative data.

The rationale for this activity is that in developing gender-sensitive projects, programmes, and policies, participants need skills to develop a focused analysis of gender issues in relation to communicable disease, and critically reflect on the strengths, weaknesses, and complementarity of a range of literature and information. For example, the readings on TB focus on evidence of sex differences in the epidemiology of TB and the possible

explanations for this; gendered influences on health-seeking behaviour with regard to TB; gender differences in access to and uptake of treatment for TB; and the socio-economic impact of TB on women or men .

This exercise raises a number of challenges. One of our aims is to illustrate the range of methodologies that can be used to explore and elucidate gender inequalities in the experience of infectious disease. We therefore include articles on the reading list that draw on both qualitative and quantitative data. It is important to stimulate participants to reflect critically on the strengths and limitations of these different methodologies in providing an understanding of gender inequalities. This is especially pertinent in a mixed group that includes participants with scientific backgrounds, who have a tendency to prioritise 'hard' quantitative data, as well as those informed by a social development background who may lack experience in handling epidemiological or health systems information.

The challenge is to demonstrate to participants the value and importance of gender-disaggregated epidemiological and health information systems data,[4] while being aware of some of the potential biases introduced by data collection processes (as illustrated by the case of gender differences in reported TB cases). Equally, it is necessary to introduce to some the value of qualitative research in enabling an understanding of *why* and *how* women's and men's experiences of disease may differ, or gender relations may affect responses to ill-health, as Nora's story illustrates. We discuss, with examples, the complementarity of qualitative and quantitative approaches, and the way in which using both approaches can facilitate a holistic understanding of the many ways gender can affect health experiences and health outcomes.

There are two difficulties here, however, which were discussed earlier in the context of the case studies. First is the lack of studies that take a comparative view of women's and men's experiences in relation to infectious disease. The majority of in-depth anthropological studies on infectious disease are 'gender blind', while a minority focus on women's experiences. Secondly, participants tend to over-generalise in their presentations on the basis of some context-specific studies. For example, participants reported that health care for women is given lower priority in the household because they are not viewed as breadwinners. However, the selected studies of care-seeking for TB present a rather more complex picture, with male breadwinners reporting an inability to complete TB treatment because of their economic responsibilities (Liefooghe 1998).

Another issue for us as course leaders is the question of how we should respond to the overview given by participants. Given that knowledge in this area is necessarily contingent and partial, it seems inappropriate to respond with a 'correct' answer. However, there is a need to counter the danger of readings being misinterpreted or taken out of context, and to respond to any technical issues or questions raised. To try to overcome this problem, we created a panel of Liverpool School of Tropical Medicine staff who are knowledgeable in these disease areas, to listen and respond to the presentations. This proved effective in stimulating debate, but it was important to avoid representing this panel as made up of experts on gender in these specific areas, due to the contextual nature of the issues discussed.

Part 2: Gender analysis and information needs

The next stage of the course aims to enable participants to conduct a gender analysis of a specific situation using some of the key concepts in contemporary discourse on gender. This involves introducing the participants to these concepts and to the available frameworks for gender analysis in health. In their working situations, participants need to produce structured analyses of specific health issues as the basis for planning. Gender analysis frameworks are useful as tools to stimulate participants to ask pertinent questions about how gender may affect the issue at hand. Participants also need to be able to identify how to collect the relevant information to allow an informed gender analysis. There is a major challenge in the tension between capturing the complexity of the ways in which gender identity potentially interacts with ill-health, and the need for participants to be confident in their role as development practitioners to make decisions on the basis of the information available.

First, participants are asked to identify the main areas that they would wish to investigate if asked to conduct a gender-sensitive analysis of a specific situation. The participants are then introduced to a gender analysis framework that has been developed by the Gender and Health Group, which appears in our 'Guidelines for the Analysis of Gender and Health'.[5] Our framework uses some core concepts central to gender analysis in development: gender divisions of labour and responsibilities; access to and control over resources; bargaining positions; and gender identities and norms. It is designed to find out how these concerns affect who gets ill (in terms of sex, age, and socio-economic status), and how individuals, households, and communities respond to ill-health. These questions are considered at the levels of the household, community, and the macro-level of states and markets. Figure 2 on page 82 shows how the framework can be used as a basis for conducting a gender analysis of primary health-care needs for Muslim communities in rural Burma.

We have found that using this framework presents several challenges for facilitators. Participants often find this matrix complex, at least initially, and feel constrained by the apparent need to fill in all the cells. They also feel the very real difficulty of making distinctions between analytical categories, such as access and control over resources, and bargaining positions. Although the matrices are intended merely to stimulate questions and identify relevant issues, participants can feel overwhelmed by the range of potential issues. We need to find ways to present the framework as a starting point, which should then stimulate a search for information in areas identified as important by participants. Prioritising areas of concern is important here, because investigating all the potential issues raised by the framework could generate unwieldy amounts of information.

Another challenge relates to the material used for analysis. It is necessary to adopt a case study to which the framework is applied. The analysis is conducted in groups to enable the sharing of ideas and insights, so a common case study is required. Participants are asked to select an area of concern (such as a specific health problem), and to conduct a gender analysis of the situation in the working and living context of *one group member*, as in the example above. This approach has the advantage of ensuring context specificity, though its success depends on the degree to which participants are able to come to a shared imagining or understanding of the specific context and the amount of relevant information possessed by the key informant on this context. An alternative is for the facilitators to provide a case study, but our experience with this approach suggests that it is difficult to provide participants with sufficient relevant information without effectively completing the exercise on their behalf.

Part 3: Ways forward – mainstreaming gender in health

This final part of the course focuses on discussion and the use of tools to stimulate reflection on how gender inequalities are produced and maintained, and therefore about the possible sites and strategies for change. Mainstreaming gender into the work and internal structure of institutions is an approach that aims to ensure that gender issues are considered throughout the policy-making, planning, and implementation processes. We feel it is our role to encourage the formulation of innovative strategies for mainstreaming gender issues into health, while aiming to keep these strategies practical and realistic.

Gender issues shape the institutions involved in health interventions in a number of ways (see Schalkwyk *et al.* 1997; UNDAW 1998 for further discussion). This has implications for policies, priorities, and practices. Organisations mirror the social structures in wider society, in that men tend to predominate in decision-making roles and senior positions, and women in caring roles. The culture and practices of institutions tend to operate on a male norm, in terms of areas such as working time, language, space, and management styles (*IDS Bulletin* 1995). This is true whether institutions are providers of health services or organisations that shape health policy and practice, such as research centres. In our own institution, men hold a large majority of senior positions.

The roles and position of women and men in health institutions, and gender stereotypes and norms in the health sector, can influence health interventions in many ways. For example, the low status of women in the health sector workforce can reinforce negative attitudes towards female clients, and the low representation of women in decision making positions can lead to male biases in priority setting.

Figure 2
Factors affecting who gets ill, northern Rakhine District, Myanmar

	Household	Communities	Influence of State and markets, international relations
Why do different groups of women and men suffer from ill-health?			
How does the ENVIRONMENT influence who becomes ill?			
How do ACTIVITIES of women and men			
How do the BARGAINING POSITIONS of women and men influence their health?	*Women and men are not able to protect their own health totally.* *Women can't make independent decisions about their health protection. Women need the permission and escort of a male family member to visit a health facility, or to ask a Burmese midwife or nurse to come over.*	*Due the cost of visiting a health facility, which most of the families can't afford, men prefer to go directly to the drug shop to get medicines for their family. The drug shop owners prescribe whatever they think is best. What kind of medicine men buy also depends on the budget they have.* *The population can't travel during the night to get health care without permission of NASAKA.* *Village leader decides who carries out forced labour, on assignment from NASAKA . Women, sick men, and more educated men are excluded. Poor men*	*have no bargaining position at all. NASAKA decides what is happening.*
How does access to and control over RESOURCES influence health of women and men?			
How do GENDER NORMS affect			

Source: Renske Wildeman, Masters in Community Health student, Liverpool School of Tropical Medicine, 2001

ERRATUM

Figure 2
Factors affecting who gets ill, northern Rakhine District, Myanmar

	Household	Communities	Influence of State and markets, international relations
Why do different groups of women and men suffer from ill-health?			
How does the ENVIRONMENT influence who becomes ill?			
How do ACTIVITIES of women and men influence their health?			
How do the BARGAINING POSITIONS of women and men influence their health?	Women and men are not able to protect their own health totally. Women can't make independent decisions about their health protection. Women need the permission and escort of a male family member to visit a health facility, or to ask a Burmese midwife or nurse to come over.	Due the cost of visiting a health facility, which most of the families can't afford, men prefer to go directly to the drug shop to get medicines for their family. The drug shop owners prescribe whatever they think is best. What kind of medicine men buy also depends on the budget they have. The population can't travel during the night to get health care without permission of NASAKA. Village leader decides who carries out forced labour, on assignment from NASAKA . Women, sick men, and more educated men are excluded. Poor men have no bargaining position at all.	NASAKA decides what is happening.
How does access to and control over RESOURCES influence health of women and men?			
How do GENDER NORMS affect responses to illness?			

Source: Renske Wildeman, Masters in Community Health student, Liverpool School of Tropical Medicine, 2001

Figure 3
SWOT analysis of MoH, Ghana

INTERNAL

Strengths

Government decentralisation policy;
District Director of Health Services (DDHS) with gender knowledge and interest;
District Health Management Team (DHMT) balanced in staff composition;
District Health Authority (DHA) has access to and power over resource use;
District Health Authority has liberty to generate and use funds;
District action planning mechanism, which has room to promote gender.

Weaknesses

Staff ability (insufficient education, skills, and experience);
No power to recruit or fire staff (centralised management);
Lack of capital resource for immediate transformation of the system, e.g. setting up of gender desk,
    gender of service provider to meet women's needs (STD clinics).

EXTERNAL

Opportunities

National and Regional support for gender training;
Regional Director interested in gender equity;
Possibility of Gender Sensitivity Programme in the district soon;
Some local NGOs promoting gender;
On-going national poverty alleviation to:
• increase women's access to resources,
• increase government interest in gender.

Threats

High staff attrition rate affects sustainable planning;
Different agendas of NGOs lead to incoherence;
Natural disasters – floods and bush fires, etc.;
Cultural and ethnic diversity poses challenges for gender analysis;
Geographical inaccessibility to some communities.

Source: Stanley Diamenu and John Koku Awoonor Williams, course participants, 2000

Conversely, the fact that women are most likely to be found in jobs which are associated with reproductive health means that men may feel uncomfortable in accessing related services, such as voluntary counselling and testing (VCT) services for HIV/AIDS.

In order to help participants to reflect on these issues, and to identify the implications for effective gender sensitive planning in participants' own working environments, we use a 'SWOT' analysis. This is a tool which will be familiar to many readers, and can be used to examine the strengths, weaknesses, opportunities, and threats of main-streaming gender within the participants' institutions. It is a useful tool for stimulating strategic and practical ideas about how to build on opportunities and address barriers. The example in Figure 3 is a SWOT analysis at different levels within the Ministry of Health (MoH) in one region of Ghana.

Each student presents her or his analysis to the plenary, to gain feedback and share ideas on ways to move from analysis to strategies for gender mainstreaming.

We found that conducting a SWOT analysis was a thought-provoking and inspiring experience for most participants, and that many of the strategies suggested were very ambitious. One participant commented: 'I learnt a lot from the SWOT exercise. I particularly remember the issue of policy evaporation.'[6] (Course evaluation 2000) The challenge for the facilitators is to encourage participants to think through the practicalities of the strategies (for example in terms of time frames, and financial and human resources) without dampening their enthusiasm.

The ultimate goal of gender analysis is to enable action to improve gender equity. Participants need to plan strategically and practically how to turn into action their reflections on their working situations. The last few days of the course are dedicated to developing, presenting, and discussing action plans. The action plan is introduced as a way to address a specific problem or situation, which builds on tools and approaches that are introduced throughout the course, such as the problem tree, frameworks for gender analysis, and SWOT analysis. Each participant produces a paper copy of their action plan, and also presents it to the group, facilitators, and some invited guests for discussion and reflection.

We found that in the presentation of the action plans, there was a tendency among some participants to avoid highlighting gender issues within all the components of the plan. The challenge for the facilitators is to provide enough individual support to each participant as they develop their plans, and to enable discussion of ways in which to incorporate a holistic gender focus without jeopardising the learning experience and feelings of ownership of the plan.

This has given rise to the idea of piloting an on-line discussion group open to all participants on future courses, once the course is completed. We hope that the group will act as a support mechanism for the participants when they return to their different working environments and begin to put their ideas into practice. One participant summarised the impact of

the course as follows: 'I see myself now as an ambassador for promoting gender equity.' (Course evaluation 2000) The course should create a supportive network, which nurtures and sustains such 'ambassadors'.

Conclusions

Teaching gender and health is an exciting, challenging, and iterative learning process. Student feedback has been invaluable in informing future directions and modifications of course content and pedagogic approaches. The process of writing this article has also been helpful in terms of thinking through how our own perspectives shape the challenges of translating an understanding of gender issues into skills for, and planning responses relevant to, participants' working situations.

Sally Theobald is a Lecturer in Social Science and International Health at the Liverpool School of Tropical Medicine, Pembroke Place, Liverpool L3 5QA.
E-mail: sjt@liv.ac.uk

Rachel Tolhurst is a Research Associate in Equity, Gender, and Health at the Liverpool School of Tropical Medicine, Pembroke Place, Liverpool L3 5QA.
E-mail: r.j.tolhurst@liv.ac.uk

Notes

1 The Gender and Health Group aims to encourage the integration and application of gender analysis into all areas of the School's work, including teaching, research, consultancy, and human resources management. Gender and Health Group members are both women and men who come from different disciplines and departments in Liverpool University and other academic institutions. For a full list of Gender and Health Group members please see our website: http://www.liv.ac.uk/lstm/gh

2 Health systems refer to the institutions that plan and provide health-care services.

3 For an example of further discussion of the management of conflict in gender training, please refer to Cousins (1988).

4 Quantitative information on disease patterns and routine information collected by health facilities, for example, on utilisation.

5 When the group formed in 1995, it felt that the existing frameworks could not grasp the complexity of gender issues involved in the planning, implementation, and evaluation of health-care provision and health research. Following an extensive literature review and sharing of experiences the group produced 'Guidelines for the Analysis of Gender and Health in Developing Countries' with the financial support of DfID (Department for International Develop-ment). These guidelines include a gender analysis framework, example of strategies for addressing gender inequalities, and case studies. They are available at http://www.liv.ac.uk/lstm/gg.html

6 'Policy evaporation' is the phenomenon of a disappearing gender focus in the move from goals or policies to specific strategies or implementation.

References

Cousins, T. (1998) 'Giving space to conflict in training', in I. Gujit and M. Shah (eds), *The Myth of Community: Gender Issues in Participatory Development*, London: Intermediate Technology Publications.

Dey, I. (1993) *Qualitative Data Analysis*, London: Routledge.

Diwan, V.K., Thorson, A., and A. Winkvist (eds) (1998) *Gender and Tuberculosis. Report from an International Research Workshop at the Nordic School of Public Health*, May 24-26, 1998, NHV Report 1998:3, Goteborg: Nordic School of Public Health.

Dolin, P. (1998) 'Tuberculosis epidemiology from a gender perspective', in V.K. Diwan, A. Thorson, and A. Winkvist (eds), *Gender and Tuberculosis. Report from an International Research Workshop at the Nordic School of Public Health*, May 24-26, 1998, NHV Report 1998:3, Goteborg: Nordic School of Public Health.

Fair, E., Islam, M.A., and S.A Chowdhury, (1998) *Tuberculosis and Gender: Treatment Seeking Behaviour and Social Beliefs of Women with Tuberculosis in Rural Bangladesh*, Working Paper no. 1, Dhaka: BRAC.

Holmes, C.B., *et al.* (1998) 'A review of sex differences in the epidemiology of tuberculosis', *International Journal of TB and Lung Disease*, 2(2): 96-104.

IDS Bulletin (1995) 'Getting institutions right for women in development', *IDS Bulletin*, 26(3).

Karim, Q. and S. Karim (1999) 'Epidemiology of HIV infection in South Africa', *AIDS*, 13(6): 4-7.

Kempkes, W. (1999) 'Community Perceptions and Practices Regarding the Provision of Care for People Living with HIV/AIDS, Chronic Illness or Disability', Masters in Community Health dissertation, Liverpool: Liverpool School of Tropical Medicine.

Liefooghe, R. (1998) 'Gender differences in beliefs and attitudes towards tuberculosis and their impact on tuberculosis control: what do we know?', in V.K. Diwan, A. Thorson, and A Winkwist (eds), *Gender and Tuberculosis. Report from an International Research Workshop at the Nordic School of Public Health*, May 24-26, 1998, NHV Report 1998:3, Goteborg: Nordic School of Public Health.

Long, V.K., Johansson, E., Lonnroth, K., Eriksson, B., Winkvist, A., and V.K. Diwan (1999) 'Longer delays in tuberculosis diagnosis among women in Vietnam', *International Journal of Tuberculosis and Lung Disease*, 3(5):388-93.

Rashed, S., Johnson, H., Dongier, P., Moreau, R., Lee, C., Crepeau, R., Lambert, J., Jefremovas, and C. Schaffer, (1999) 'Determinants of the Permethrin impregnated bed nets (PIB) in the Republic of Benin: the role of women in the acquisition and utilisation of PIBs', *Social Science and Medicine*, 49: 993-1005.

Schalkwyk, J., Woroniuk, B., and H. Thomas (1997) *Handbook for Mainstreaming: a Gender Perspective in the Health Sector*, Stockholm: Department for Democracy and Social Development, Health Division, Sida (Swedish International Development Co-operation Agency).

Zeirler, S. and N. Krieger (1997) 'Reframing women's risk: social inequalities and HIV infection', *Annual Review of Public Health*, 18: 401-36.

UNDAW (1998) 'Women and Health: Mainstreaming the Gender Perspective into the Health Sector', report of the Expert Group Meeting, 28 September – 2 October 1998, Tunis.

Attitudes towards abortion among medical trainees in Mexico City public hospitals

Deyanira González de León Aguirre and Deborah L. Billings

During the past decade, there has been considerable discussion in Mexico about abortion, and some progress has been made in improving legislation in line with agreements made at the International Conference on Population and Development (ICPD) held in Cairo in 1994. The attitude of physicians toward abortion is a topic of interest throughout the world. In particular, this due to the fact that in many places physicians play the role of gatekeeper, controlling women's access to safe abortion services. This article explores the attitudes among medical residents[1] in obstetrics and gynaecology in Mexico City regarding abortion. Most residents accept that abortion services should be provided to women who become pregnant as a result of rape; to women for whom pregnancy could be life-threatening; or in case of severe foetal malformation. The majority believed that public health systems should offer abortion services for legal indications. However, few of the medical professionals interviewed said that they would personally provide abortion services.

Historically, the debate about abortion has focused on two irreconcilable positions — those who are in favour of a woman's right to choose, and those who are against abortion. This approach has impeded discussion about the true dimensions of the problem. In Mexico, unsafe abortion is the fourth most important cause of maternal mortality (Lezana 1999). An estimated one out of every three women experiencing abortion requires hospitalisation for emergency care (López García 1994). However, in Mexico as elsewhere in the world, women who find it most difficult to gain access to emergency care have a greater risk of dying or suffering from short- and long-term health consequences than women whose access to emergency services is more immediate (Maine 1997). An analysis of maternal mortality in Mexico by Lozano *et al.* (1994) demonstrates that women living in highly marginalised areas are twice as likely to die from abortion complications, relative to women living in regions that are not marginalised.[2]

The International Conference on Population and Development (ICPD) in 1994 was the first global forum where agreement was reached firstly that unsafe abortion must be recognised and addressed as a public health problem. During the five-year review of ICPD implementation, governments reaffirmed their commitment and called for health systems to make services accessible to women, stating, '...In circumstances where abortion is not against the law, health systems should train and equip health-service providers and should take other measures to ensure that such abortion is safe and accessible. Additional measures should be taken to safeguard women's health.' (UN General Assembly 1999, para. 63(iii))

Abortion has been widely recognised as an important social and public health problem in Mexico. However, since the 1970s, commentators from the most conservative of religious and political circles have generated confusion and misinformation about abortion. They have blocked debate on initiatives to update existing laws, presented at different key moments by women's groups linked to the feminist movement and by certain actors within the government. The majority of legislators, political leaders of different affiliations, and health care authorities have evaded the responsibility of discussing the repercussions of existing abortion legislation, which favours and fosters the clandestine practice of abortion. Such practices result in a high number of women dying from unsafely performed abortions or suffering from complications that could have been prevented (Langer 1999; Tarrés 1993).[3]

In recent years, however, political life in Mexico has been marked by significant change, and the public has been involved increasingly in the discussion of national problems. Academic and non-governmental organisations have intensified their struggle for the recognition of sexual and reproductive rights and to support women's abilities to exercise these rights. Their work has made the complex issue of abortion more visible, in part through new initiatives to modify existing laws. Interest on the part of distinct sectors of society in the problem of abortion has increased over the years, as has the level of public discussion. Public opinion polls indicate that 83·5 per cent of the Mexican population believes that the decision to interrupt a pregnancy should reside with women and their partners (GIRE 1998; Population Council 2001). Particular cases have come to pubic attention: for example, in 1999 in Mexicali, Baja California, health authorities in a public hospital denied legal abortion services to 13-year-old Paulina del Carmen Ramírez Jacinto, who had been

raped. In the following year in the state of Guanajuato, the local Congress approved a legal initiative to outlaw abortion in cases of rape (Lamas and Bissell 2000; Poniatowska 2000). The arguments of those who defended the idea of life from the moment of conception and who supported more restrictive laws were severely questioned by the public. The media dedicated significant space to the discussion of these occurrences, and the abortion issue divided positions of the leaders within the conservative National Action Party (PAN), which won the presidential election in July 2000, and currently governs in the states of Guanajuato and Baja California. In the case of the reform in Guanajuato, the local governor was pressured to carry out a public opinion poll that showed over-whelming opposition to a change in the law. Subsequently, he vetoed the new legislation, and abortion remains legal in cases of pregnancy as a result of rape in the state of Guanajuato (Lamas and Bissell 2000).

Concurrently, in mid-August 2000, the interim Mayor of Mexico City, Rosario Robles, presented a bill to broaden the bases on which legal abortion could be obtained in Mexico City. Existing legislation did not penalise abortion performed for the following indications: to terminate pregnancy as the result of rape; to save the life of the pregnant woman; or in cases of pregnancy resulting from an accident beyond the woman's control. The bill was passed by a majority in the Federal District Legislative Assembly (ALDF), and added three more indications for which abortion would not be penalized: when the pregnancy presents grave risk to the health of the woman; in the case of severe congenital foetal malformation; and in the case of artificial insemination performed without the consent of the woman. In addition, the legislation defined the responsibilities of the judicial and health sectors, including physicians, in the provision of abortion services, and the steps that need to be followed to ensure women's access to safe abortion services in the case of rape or artificial insemination without consent (Asamblea Legislativa del Distrito Federal 2000; Lamas and Bissell 2000; Ortega Ortiz 2000). Such procedures are notably absent from legislation in most Mexican states, presenting important barriers to women's access to safe services.

Physicians' role in abortion care services in Mexico City

The new legislation in Mexico City provides a broadened framework for the practice of legal abortion, and the responsibilities set forth in the legislative procedures are relevant to all health-care providers, including medical residents in obstetrics and gynaecology. In addition, international agreements to which Mexico is a signatory provide additional weight to the importance of training medical professionals in abortion care.

Specific responsibilities of physicians are explicitly defined in the revised penal code of Mexico City, which states that physicians must provide pregnant women with objective, truthful, sufficient, and opportune information about the abortion procedure, including its risks, consequences, and effects. They must also provide information about support and alternatives, so that a woman can make her decision in a free, informed, and responsible manner. Information should be provided to the woman immediately, and the physician should not attempt to influence or delay the decision of the woman. In the case of rape, the local Justice Department must authorise the abortion procedure within 24 hours of the woman reporting the rape, and public health institutions must confirm the pregnancy and provide the abortion service when the woman requests this procedure (Asamblea Legislativa del Distrito Federal 2000). Such modifications are significant in

facilitating women's access to safe and legal abortion services, given the numerous delays in processes often experienced by women seeking abortion in case of rape.

Attitudes of physicians towards abortion

Studies from many different countries, particularly the United States, Canada, and from various European countries, indicate general patterns in the attitudes of physicians toward abortion. Within the health profession, those specialising in obstetrics and gynaecology tend to be among the most conservative in their attitudes; young professionals tend to be more cautious in their practice; and women physicians tend to be more willing to provide abortion services under a wider range of circumstances. Those identifying themselves as practising Catholics tend to express moral and religious opposition to abortion.

Conscientious objection clauses that appear in the legislation of some countries enable health-care professionals to abstain from providing this basic health service to women, because of their moral or religious beliefs. However, they do not exempt health-care institutions or systems from offering safe abortion services, if these are legal. In some countries where legislation allows for the practice of abortion under limited circumstances, the opinion of two or more physicians is needed before the abortion can be authorised. In contexts where few qualified physicians exist, or where few physicians support and are trained to provide safe abortion services, this creates even greater barriers for women who need to access abortion services. Where legislation permits abortion for a variety of indications, more than 90 per cent are performed during the first trimester of pregnancy. Many physicians do not oppose abortion during this time period or in situations of grave risk to the woman's health or life and foetal malformation. However, physicians' attitudes shift significantly when asked about abortion during more advanced stages of pregnancy, or for reasons that are social rather than health-related (Cook 1991; David 1992).

Another significant factor influencing the attitude of physicians toward abortion is their professional training. In the case of the USA, for example, abortion is one of the most commonly performed surgical procedures, with between 1.2 and 1.5 million procedures per year (Rosenfield 1999). Yet numerous authors have documented the substantial decrease in the number of trained physicians willing to provide abortion services, as well as the concentration of available services, with nine in ten abortion service providers located in metropolitan areas. Few obstetrics, gynaecology, or family medicine departments include first trimester abortion in their routine activities.[4] In the majority of cases, training is optional, and is conducted outside of teaching hospitals in clinics such as those belonging to Planned Parenthood (Castle and Hakim-Elahi 1996). In general, physicians providing abortion services are often stigmatised by their colleagues and many consider that learning the skills necessary for abortion are of little use for their professional development and prestige. Yet, at the same time some physicians train in abortion management, in order to be able to increase their earnings in their private practice (Scully 1994).

Attitudes of medical residents towards abortion

Over the past ten years in Mexico, eminent health-care professionals have contributed to an analysis of the social and public health consequences of unsafe abortion, giving weight to the movement to modify restrictive abortion laws throughout the country.

In Mexico abortion legislation is defined at state level; thus the 31 states plus the capital, Mexico City, have independent and differing legislation. Throughout the country, abortion is legal for women whose pregnancy is the result of rape. However, providers are often unwilling to perform the procedure and women's access to services in the public sector is very limited. The majority of physicians in Mexico take a conservative stance on the issue of abortion, and have remained at the margins of public debate on the topic.

In general, physicians in Mexico who refuse to perform abortions do so because the practice is against their religious beliefs or because of their lack of knowledge about existing laws which provide for legal abortions under varying circumstances. On the other hand, neither moral condemnation nor the threat of legal penalties has impeded the practice of abortion in private clinics throughout the country, through which physicians generate significant earnings. Relatively few physicians state that they provide abortion services because of an ethical commitment to women who request the service (González de León 1999).

Casanueva and colleagues (1997) focused on 193 specialists who work in public hospitals in Mexico City. The specialists worked in different areas, as internists,[5] paediatricians, gynae-cologists, and neurologists. The study found that over half (59 per cent) were in agreement with abortion in case of foetal malformation. This increased to 91 per cent in cases of severe malformation, where the newborn would die outside the womb. In contrast, only 15 per cent were in agreement with abortion on demand, and gynaecologists and neurologists favoured this the least. Physicians stating that they did not practise religion, and those over the age of 35, were generally more supportive of abortion.

One obstacle to a comprehensive understanding of abortion by doctors is the lack of sexual and reproductive health content in medical education. Most medical school programmes frame their teaching using biomedical and curative models of health, which offer future health-care professionals few practical elements needed to understand and apply concepts of sexual and reproductive health. The emphasis on ethics, generally approached from a conservative moral-religious perspective that includes abstract values about human life, has a significant influence on the presentation of abortion in medical school programmes. In university classrooms and health services, it is not uncommon to witness abortion presented as a moral rather than a public health issue, and induced abortion referred to as 'criminal abortion', associated with murder and infanticide. In addition, the legal aspects of abortion are not adequately presented in most medical schools, and few professionals understand the laws that regulate and allow for its practice.

In order to better understand the attitudes toward abortion of medical residents in obstetrics and gynaecology practising in public hospitals in Mexico City, a study was conducted between February and April 2000 (González de León Aguirre and Salinas Urbina 2000), based on self-administered closed-ended questionnaires applied to 121 medical residents working in seven public hospitals in Mexico City.[6] Most (89 per cent) of the respondents were between 23–30 years of age; 98 per cent were Mexican citizens; 61 per cent were single; and 71 per cent had no children. The sample was almost evenly divided between men and women: 54 per cent men, and 48 per cent women. The majority were studying at a public university (81 per cent), with almost half (49 per cent) attending the National Autonomous University of Mexico (UNAM). Eighty-nine percent identified themselves as Catholic, with 70 per cent noting sporadic attendance at religious services (during special events, or about once a month).

Only 64 percent of the medical residents surveyed knew that abortion is legal for some indications in Mexico City. Most (75 per cent) believed that women seek abortions because of a lack of education about sexuality and information about contraceptive methods. Twenty-four percent noted that women themselves should be responsible for making the decision about having an abortion; 21 per cent thought that women together with their partner should make the decision; and 27 per cent thought that women together with their partner and physician should make the decision. Only 2 percent indicated that the physician should be responsible for the decision to have an abortion while 15 percent responded that women should not abort and thus there should be no decision-making process.

Medical residents were asked about different indications for which they would accept the decision to abort. The results are shown in Table 1. It is clear from the responses that the majority of residents included in the study generally accept abortion for the indications included in the current Mexico City legislation, with a distinction being made in terms of the severity of the foetal malformation. That is, significantly more medical residents accepted the decision to abort in case of severe malformations making extra-uterine life impossible, as compared to those accepting abortion in case of fetal malformation compatible with life outside of the uterus. However, abortion for reasons related to women's choice or socio-economic conditions was generally opposed by the medical residents included in the study.

Table 1.

Percentage distribution of obstetric-gynaecologist residents' acceptance of abortion under distinctive indications

INDICATION	ACCEPT (%)	OPPOSE (%)	NOT SURE (%)
Fetal malformation incompatible with extra-uterine life	94	4	2
Pregnancy poses risk to the life of the woman	91	6	3
Pregnancy resulting from rape	89	7	4
Woman has severe heart condition	59	32	9
Woman has AIDS or is HIV-positive	52	36	12
Fetal malformation compatible with extra-uterine life	48	35	17
Woman with psychological problems or with risk of psychological problems because of the pregnancy	26	61	13
Woman or partner with poor socio-economic conditions	19	73	8
Women, married or single, who does not want to be pregnant	15	82	3
Woman with children whose spouse died or abandoned family	12	81	7
Adolescent without the means to support a family	12	81	7
Contraceptive method failure	11	81	8
Woman who is studying and cannot attend to a child	8	85	7

A final general question posed to medical residents was to ask what they would do if a woman asked for helped in interrupting her pregnancy. The reason for the abortion was not defined in the question. Forty-eight per cent responded that they would not perform the abortion, nor would they refer the woman to another physician; 28 per cent would not perform the abortion but would refer the woman to another doctor; just 5 per cent noted that they would perform the abortion; 10 per cent responded that it would depend on the situation; and 9 per cent responded that they did not know. Thus, while attitudes are fairly open towards abortion among residents in obstetrics and gynaecology, depending on the situation of the woman, few of those surveyed stated that they would actually provide the service, with 10 per cent clarifying that it would depend on the situation of the woman. Yet three-quarters of all respondents noted that public health institutions should offer abortion services for the indications permitted by law.

The question remains, who will provide the services?

In summary, the results from this study highlight that medical residents preparing for a speciality in obstetrics and gynaecology accept a woman's or couple's decision to have an abortion under a limited set of circumstances, but very few are willing to provide the service to women. These data, combined with findings from other studies, indicate the need to introduce substantial changes in medical school programmes, so that they include more precise information about reproductive and sexual health and abortion from a public health perspective, and to promote a broader debate about abortion in medical schools, health services, and medical associations. One area of urgent action is the development of strategies that create new ethical positions and perspectives among physicians on the issue of abortion.

Abortion is a complex issue that is being approached increasingly as a priority area within public health at state and national levels in Mexico. It is a problem that is faced every day by many Mexican women. No woman should have to suffer the physical or emotional consequences of, nor fear the risk of death from, an unsafe abortion. The viability of the reforms in abortion legislation in Mexico City depends in large part on the ability of local legislators to continue the open and honest discussion about abortion and the willingness of health-care professionals to fully implement new laws.

Experience throughout the world has shown that the position taken by the medical community on abortion plays a central role in the application of laws regulating abortion and therefore women's access to safe services. Thus, without the support of physicians, the reach and impact of the reforms passed in the Federal District and in all of the Mexican states will be very limited.

Deyanira González de León Aguirre is Associate Professor at Universidad Autónoma Metropolitana Xochimilco, Departamento de Atención a la Salud, Calzada del Hueso #1100, Delegación Coyoacan, CP 04960, México DF, México.
E-mail: *deyagla@yahoo.com.mx*

Deborah L. Billings is Senior Research Associate at Ipas, Campeche 280 Oficina 601, Colonia Hipodromo Condesa, CP 06100, México DF, México.
E-mail: *dbillings@webtelmex.net.mx*

Notes

1 Medical residents are post-graduate students who are undergoing clinical training in a speciality, such as obstetrics and gynaecology. Residents are usually paid during this period of their training.

2 The index of marginalisation is based on variables including housing conditions, level of education, and the presence of indigenous populations. The researchers categorised marginalisation into four levels: low, medium, high, and very high.

3 The World Health Organisation defines unsafe abortion as the termination of pregnancy by persons lacking necessary skills or in an environment lacking minimal standards or both.

4 First trimester refers to the first three months of pregnancy.

5 Internists are physicians who have completed their residency in internal medicine. They attend to many different types of patients but do not have training in paediatrics, gynaecology, or psychiatry.

6 The hospitals in the survey were drawn from the following health care systems: the Ministry of Health (SSA) (one hospital); the Ministry of Health of the Federal District (SSADF) (three hospitals); the Social Security and Services Institute for State Workers (ISSSTE) (two hospitals); and the Mexican Institute of Social Security (IMSS) (one hospital).

References

Asamblea Legislativa del Distrito Federal (2000) 'Decreto por el que se reforman y adicionan diversas disposiciones del código penal para del Distrito Federal y del código de procedimientos penales para del Distrito Federal', *Gaceta Oficial del Distrito Federal*, 148.

Casanueva, E., Lisker, R., Carnevale, A., and E. Alonso (1997) 'Attitudes of Mexican physicians toward induced abortion', *International Journal of Gynecology and Obstetrics*, 56.

Castle, M.A. and E. Hakim-Elahi (1996) 'Abortion education for residents', *Obstetrics and Gynecology*, 87(4).

Cook, R.J. (1991) 'Leyes y políticas sobre el aborto: retos y oportunidades', *Debate Feminista (México)*, 1.

David, H.P. (1992) 'Abortion in Europe 1920-1991: A public health perspective', *Studies in Family Planning*, 23(1).

GIRE (1998) *Boletín Trimestral sobre Reproducción Elegida*, 17.

González de Leon Aguirre, D. and A.A. Salinas Urbina (2000) *Resultados de una encuesta sobre aborto aplicada a residentes de la especialidad en ginecología y obstetricia en hospitales públicos de la Ciudad de México, Reporte de Investigación No. 89*, México City: UAM.

González de Leon, D. (1999) 'Una mirada a la situación del aborto en México', in L. Scavone (ed.), *Género y salud reproductiva en América Latina*, Cartago, Costa Rica: Libro Universitario Regional.

Lamas, M. and S. Bissell (2000) 'Abortion and politics in Mexico: "Context is all"', *Reproductive Health Matters*, 8(16).

Langer, A. (1999) 'Planificación familiar y salud reproductiva o planificación familiar vs. salud reproductiva', in M. Bronfman and R. Castro (eds), *Salud, cambio social y políticas. Perspectivas desde América Latina*, Mexico City: Edamex/ Instituto Nacional de Salud Pública.

Lezana, M.A. (1999) 'Evolución de las tasas de mortalidad materna en México', in Ma. del Carmen Elu and Elsa Santos Pruneda (eds), *Una nueva mirada a la mortalidad materna en México*, Mexico City: UNFPA/ Population Council.

López García, R. (1994) 'El aborto como problema de salud pública', in Ma. del Carmen Elu and Ana Langer (eds), *Maternidad sin riesgos en México*, Mexico City: IMES.

Lozano, R., Hernández, B., and A. Langer, (1994) 'Factores sociales y económicos de la mortalidad materna en México', in Ma. del Carmen Elu and Ana Langer (eds), *Maternidad sin riesgos en México*, Mexico City: IMES.

Maine, D. (ed.) (1997) *Prevention of Maternal Mortality: Supplement to the International Journal of Gynecology and Obstetrics*, 59 (supplement 2).

Ortega Ortiz, A. (2000) 'El aborto legal en México', paper for workshop, 'Taller de capacitación jurídica legal para trabajadores del sector salud y otras instancias involucradas respeto a la interrupción legal del emabarazo', September 21-2, Mexico City.

Poniatowska, E. (2000) *Las mil y una... (la herida de Paulina)*, Mexico: Plaza y Janés Editores.

Population Council (2001) 'National Survey about Abortion in Mexico', unpublished, New York: Population Council.

Rosenfield, A. (1999) 'Foreword', in M. Paul, *et al.* (eds), *A Clinician's Guide to Medical and Surgical Abortion*, New York: Churchill/ Livingstone.

Scully, D. (1994) *Men who Control Women's Health. The Mis-education of Obstetrician-Gynecologists*, New York: Teachers College Press, Columbia University.

Tarrés M.L. (1993) 'El movimiento de mujeres y el sistema político mexicano: análisis de la lucha por la liberalización del aborto. 1976-1990', *Estudios Sociológicos*, 60(32).

UN General Assembly (1999) *Key Actions for the Future Implementation of the Programme of Action of the ICPD*, UN General Assembly June 1999.

Enhancing gender equity in health programmes:
monitoring and evaluation

Mohga Kamal Smith

This article argues for the need to conduct monitoring and evaluation in health programmes and advocacy in a gender-sensitive way, to ensure that interventions fulfil their goal of improving public health, have a beneficial impact on women and on gender relations, and contribute towards human health and poverty eradication.

'Why should we waste time and money to get separate information? Are you telling me that girls have more diarrhoea than boys?'
(Researcher collecting baseline information for a health project in Africa)

Over the past ten years there has been increasing international recognition of the vital role to be played by investment in health care in the poverty-reduction strategies supported by governments and international donors. Parallel to this, there has been a growing debate at national level on the need for gender analysis in mainstream health programming and policy (Standing 2000). Previously, concern for women's and gender issues was confined to a narrow focus on women's reproductive role, and hence on mother-and-child services, rather than taking account of women's needs, caring roles, and access and utilisation of health services.[1] Gender-sensitive monitoring and evaluation is an essential component of this new agenda. It is a key principle in gender work to question any

assumptions that a particular project or programme reaches all members of a community and has a similar impact on all of them.

Since the 1970s, feminist research in many different countries in both the North and the South has shown the negative impact on women, their families, and communities of focusing development projects and programmes on the 'household', 'family', or 'community'. Using these units of analysis conceals the power relations, potential conflicts of interest, and differing roles and responsibilities of individuals. A policy or a project that is judged to have improved the welfare of the household may not have affected all household members positively, or equally. It may even exacerbate gender inequity. In the health sector, for example, family-planning projects have targeted women as primary users and beneficiaries of family-planning services, because the methods they promote are predominantly used by women (Hartmann 1987). However, this approach is ineffective because, first, women are not often the decision makers on fertility issues, since unequal gender relations in the household enable men to control women's sexuality and fertility. Second, targeting women in family planning means that men's role in sexual health and reproduction has been largely overlooked. Monitoring of a family-planning project in Ethiopia revealed that the focus on women precluded any reference to condom use, despite the rise in HIV/AIDS in the country and women's vulnerability to the infection (internal Oxfam report 1995). The evaluation led the NGO to adopt condom promotion as one of its strategies.

Gender-blind health programmes have also been responsible for health professionals taking for granted existing male/female power relations and divisions of labour, rather than challenging attitudes in the community about them. This not only means that programmes may fail, but also runs the risk of worsening women's position in the household or community. For example, the fact that many health professionals take the caring role of women for granted means that mothers can be blamed for children's illnesses or malnutrition, which may bring reprisals, especially if the sick child was a boy. Thus, blaming women will not only fail to improve the child's health, but can also worsen the situation of women at home. Another example of how ignoring gender relations can lead to projects failing arises from the practice of growth monitoring, which has been promoted for the last three decades as a simple intervention to improve children's nutrition by monitoring changes in their weight in relation to their age or height. Programmes focusing on growth monitoring were also intended to empower women, through providing them with knowledge about nutrition and child growth, and by involving them in the actual monitoring. However, it is now well recognised that many of the crucial causes of malnutrition which influence child growth go beyond women's sphere of control. In addition, assessments of the impact on women of participating in growth-monitoring programmes have shown that in fact it can be a significant additional demand on women's time and workload (Smith 1997). The impact of policies and programmes on various sections in society needs to be disaggregated, bearing in mind gender and other social relations.

However, even if gender is taken into account as a differentiating factor in programming, this aspect of social differentiation is rarely seen in relation to other aspects. Thus disabled or older women, or women from minority groups, are not often taken into account when designing policies or projects, and hence they do not feature in monitoring and evaluation data. Young or adolescent girls may be affected by the same intervention in different ways from other women or from men. Urban women may have different gender roles or tasks than do rural women.

For example, in an urban health project in Yemen, women in the targeted communities were working as street sweepers. The project staff did not initially appreciate that women's heavy and time-consuming workload was the reason why they preferred to bottle-feed their infants. Therefore staff targeted messages at women, promoting breast-feeding and growth-monitoring, and discouraging bottle-feeding. Project evaluation and studies of women's health and the overall social influences on health of the community revealed some basic problems facing the women. They included the fact that women had no means of taking maternity leave from street-sweeping after delivery, and the fact that they had to spend time begging, which meant they were away from their children for long periods. The project worked with a garbage-collection scheme which was operating in the same area to develop a system to enable women to attain their legal entitlements regarding sick leave and maternity leave. At the same time, the health-education component of the project underwent changes to accommodate the realities of women's lives.

Monitoring and evaluation in health programming

Monitoring refers to the systematic and regular gathering of information about the progress of a development programme or project, the implementation of organisational procedures, or changes to the policy environment. The aim of monitoring is to ensure that goals are met, by highlighting any changes that need to be made to policy or practice. In contrast, *evaluation* is an assessment of a project or programme, or of a policy or organisational performance, against stated objectives and expectations at a given point in time.

As development agencies have got better at assessing their impact and improving their analysis, the application of gender analysis to monitoring and evaluation has increasingly been acknowledged to be an essential part of this process (Roche 1999). Monitoring and evaluation in health programming is now moving away from measuring the effects of projects and programmes on the 'household', 'family', or 'community', to gender-sensitive monitoring and evaluation, an essential component of a health-promotion strategy.

Policy monitoring for advocacy purposes

Policy monitoring aims to collect information to measure the impact of policies in relation to their stated objectives. Monitoring can be used to challenge bad policies and engage in advocacy on behalf of those affected negatively by such policies. Policy monitoring can be an empowering process for women and men, enabling them to express their views to policy makers. There are numerous studies of the impact of health policies such as user

fees and health-sector reforms on the access of poor women and men to services. Often these policies have been implemented in the absence of monitoring systems to measure the process of implementation as well as their effects, which would identify the scope for modifications or changes. (See Standing 1997 for a more detailed analysis of health-sector reform policy from a gender perspective.)

Health-policy monitoring can enable policy-makers and interested groups to examine systematically and regularly both the process and impact of turning a certain policy into reality. This enables health policy-makers to intervene and make necessary changes to such a policy, in order to achieve its overall aim. Gender-sensitive health-policy monitoring can enable civil society, including women's organisations and groups, systematically to gather data to influence policy-makers in favour of gender-equitable health policies. Both women and men within communities can also be empowered through methods of participatory policy monitoring to voice their opinions and raise their concerns on policies which have a negative impact on them.

An example of gender-sensitive health-policy monitoring is the focus on user fees, introduced in many sub-Saharan African countries in the 1980s and 1990s, as a result of IMF/World Bank Structural Adjustment Policies which encouraged cut-backs on social spending. Monitoring the impact of user fees illustrates clearly how gender identity has an effect on access to medical care. In general, user fees have had very serious effects on poor people's access to health services (Gilson 1997). However, these effects are not the same for men and women: although it may be the case that all poor people have difficulty using health services for which they have to pay, attention to gender perspectives reveals specific gender-related issues.

Oxfam research on access to health services in Uganda reveals the way in which the impact of user fees on people's use of health services varies according to gender (Oxfam unpublished report 1998). Men tended to seek treatment for sexually transmitted diseases (STDs) in private clinics, or by buying medicines from drug shops. They reported that they chose these forms of treatment because they trusted them, and had the money to pay for them. Adolescent boys' main reason for using the same services was the fact that the shops were perceived as preserving confidentiality, in comparison with other methods of treatment. In contrast, women were particularly late in seeking treatment, partly because of the low priority that they placed on their own health needs. When they did seek treatment, they used traditional healers, rather than going to private clinics or shops; they said that this was partly for financial reasons. In addition, women feared stigma if they used the services of clinics to treat STDs. Adolescent girls went nowhere, ascribing their failure to seek treatment to the risk of stigma and the unaffordable costs. It was clear from the research that the rising cost of medicines after user fees were introduced further deterred people from accessing formal medical treatment, and compounded existing obstacles created by poverty and by discrimination linked to gender and other aspects of social identity.

Gender-sensitive health-policy monitoring has also shown that user fees have a negative impact on women as carers. When patients do not use health services, they are cared for by others in the household, usually women. Therefore, care for the sick increases the workload of women. In addition, studies demonstrate that imposing (or increasing) charges for health services leads to a heavier work burden for women who earn income outside the home, who have to work even harder and longer hours to raise money to pay for care (Moser, no date). The effects of increased workloads on women spill over to the daughters who assume their mother's caring role, often at the expense of their schooling. It is clear from this that, in order to use health-policy monitoring to enhance gender equity, not only do data have to be differentiated in terms of women and men in various groups, but it is important to take into account the different status, roles, and responsibilities of women and men, as well as their differing degrees of participation in decision-making processes.

The sorts of question which need to be asked in gender-sensitive health-policy monitoring include the following:

- Given the role of women as carers/health-care providers, how will the health policy in question affect that role?
- Given that less priority is attached to the importance of women using services, and that some women attach less priority to using services themselves, what effects will the policy have in exacerbating or balancing this inequity?
- How does the health policy affect the participation of women and men in decision making regarding health care at the various levels: household, local, and national?

In addition, gender-analysis frameworks used in project planning, monitoring, and evaluation, for example the Harvard framework, can be used (see March *et al.* 1999 for more information on such frameworks). Gender-specific frameworks enable the development of gendered monitoring and evaluation systems, and some of these frameworks have been applied to health projects (ibid.).

A gender-sensitive monitoring exercise focusing on the Assuit Burns Centre, a health project in Upper Egypt, provided an in-depth understanding of the gender dimensions of burns in a poor rural area of Upper Egypt, revealing women's particular vulnerability to burns, and their lack of access to health services. The Burns Centre is supported by Oxfam GB, which sees it as an innovative project addressing women's specific needs, which recognises that gender roles affect women's physical and psychological health and social well-being. Although it began as a curative/ rehabilitative service, the Burns Centre subsequently expanded its functions to community-based activities in local villages. It takes a comprehensive approach to burns, integrating preventive, curative, and rehabilitative aspects of primary health care, and recognising that understanding the gender dimensions of the problem of burns is crucial in ensuring that women receive proper support. Women's access to the Burns Centre, as to any other health service, is determined by many factors: the perceived need for health care, the decision to go and use the service, the service available, and the costs of care, including travelling and lost income opportunities.

In the monitoring exercise, the example of one woman, Hodda, was given. Hodda was cooking a meal for her family when the stove fell on the ground, and her face and arms got burnt. A gender analysis of burns in Upper Egypt tells us that it is usually women who are affected by burns, while they are performing their domestic tasks of cooking and baking. In the Burns Centre, Hodda received treatment and care. Her disfigured face and incapacitated arms needed many sessions of rehabilitation, in addition to an operation. Although the physical complications of burns, such as disfigurement and disability, are the same for women and men, the social complications are different. Disfigured women have to face many prejudices which affect their social lives. For example, unmarried women who are burned may never get married, and may live almost as outcasts from society, which demands conformity to gendered expectations of female beauty and capacity for physical work. The Burns Centre provides a high-

quality health-care service which considers those factors. For example, a relative (usually the husband or brother) is taught basic rehabilitation skills, jointly with the woman. Work with schools and community workers tries to raise awareness about preventive measures and about the need for immediate treatment of burns. A health-education programme in schools has galvanised teachers, parents, and pupils into raising awareness and taking preventive measures.

Why monitor health projects, and for whom?

Earlier sections have explained why it is crucial to ensure that gender analysis is a core component of monitoring of health projects. However, each monitoring process is catalysed by its own short-term goals and intentions. In the health sector and beyond, the immediate aims of monitoring can range from a focus on the number and satisfaction of users, to the need to satisfy a donor that its funds have been well spent and are having a positive impact on the problem that the project was set up to address. There are usually several linked motives behind a monitoring process.

To return to the example of the Assuit Burns Centre: monitoring and evaluation were done regularly to satisfy many actors. Oxfam GB, as a donor, wanted good reasons to justify its support for a service which was relatively expensive, and curative rather than preventive (contrary to the prevailing view that curative services are the responsibility of governments, and that NGOs should focus on prevention). The partner group which implemented the project consisted of a dedicated plastic surgeon, foreign nationals, and relatives of some patients. They required monitoring and evaluation as a means of helping them to prove the impact of the project, and hence to raise funds sufficient to sustain the Centre and implement other activities. Oxfam and the partner group shared the common goal of wanting to find cost-effective ways of addressing the problems of burns in a comprehensive way, to ensure the sustainability of the project itself, and justify Oxfam's support.

A summary of the reasons for monitoring health-care projects is given in Table 1.

When should health projects be monitored?

Some development literature refers to monitoring as one step in the 'project cycle'. This implies that monitoring takes place during the implementation phase of the project only. However, if necessary changes are to be introduced into the project, and if projects are to foster learning by findings being fed into policy processes and organisational development, a different model of monitoring needs to be adopted. The preoccupation with the project cycle needs to be challenged. Instead, we need to envisage monitoring as a process which goes on throughout the entire life of a project and beyond. In this way we can create an opportunity for continuous learning.

Who should monitor and evaluate health projects?

In the case of health projects run by NGOs, it is most usual for project staff to monitor the performance of the project, through visits and discussions with partners and implementing agencies. There are advantages in involving staff in monitoring the performance of the project. After all, they know the project context and activities well, and can identify their strengths and weaknesses, and opportunities for improvement. They are also in a position to recognise positive and negative changes in the health of community members. However, there are also potential pitfalls. For example, staff are often too busy to document monitoring visits/discussions accessibly, to allow data to be shared and to enhance learning. Training in participatory methods of monitoring and evaluation could help staff to collect, analyse, and present data on changes in the project area. Of course, the involvement of 'the community' is not an automatic guarantee of a gender-sensitive perspective in the monitoring process. Community leaders, usually men, may see the benefits of projects in different ways from the women in the community. Local knowledge of project and context does not automatically translate to knowledge of gender concerns and commitment to ensuring that these are included within the project, or within the monitoring or evaluation process.

Table 1: Aims of health-care project monitoring

Why?	For whom?
Efficient use of resources	Managers, staff, funders
Input into planning and adjusting strategies	Managers, staff, 'community'
To identify opportunities	Managers, staff
To identify problems and enable solutions	Managers, staff, 'community'
Accountability to different stakeholders	Managers, staff, 'community', funders
Documentation for evaluations and impact-assessment studies	Managers, staff, 'community', funders
Knowledge and learning	Staff, other interested groups, managers
Empowering people to take action	'Community'

For example, men may judge projects which offer care for mothers and children as adequate for addressing women's health needs. However, in some cases such projects may ignore the needs and perceptions of women whose health concerns are not connected with child-bearing or rearing, such as adolescents, older women, or women of reproductive age who do not have children. It is also important to recognise that, especially on the topic of health, women and men may prefer to talk to someone of their own sex. For example, a refugee camp in south Sudan was visited by many outsiders. Only when an Oxfam GB female gender adviser with a health background went to talk to young girls was their need for cloth to make sanitary towels identified (personal communication). The young women had been too shy to ask the male aid workers, and none of the latter had thought of asking.

To counter such problems, training is needed in gender analysis for all those involved in monitoring and evaluation. In the Burns Centre project, monitoring was done by project staff (men and women) in regular dialogue with Oxfam. Staff visited the project villages and held discussions with various members of the village, including women, during home visits. However, the project did not have an explicit gender-monitoring framework, and documentation of the monitoring process was not always adequate.

What needs to be monitored?

Monitoring is usually restricted to the objectives of a project, which often rely on two main elements. The first of these is SMART (specific, measurable, attainable, relevant, and time-bound) objectives. The second of these elements is baseline data on the context of the project and the community in the project area. Baseline data are essential if changes are to be measured; but despite this, in many cases, projects are initiated with minimal baseline data – whether secondary or primary data.

It is common sense to say that in order to design gender-specific monitoring systems, at the very least the project objectives and baseline data collected at the planning stage must be disaggregated by sex. Objectives should recognise gender roles and responsibilities, and women's and men's differing degrees of access to resources, information, and services. Detailed baseline information is needed; superficial information on gender issues may lead a project to misfire. For example, when designing a project with the objective of reducing the incidence of schistosomiasis (bilharzia), a belief that men are most at risk because they work in fields where they are exposed to irrigation water may lead to their being targeted in particular. However, women may also be in the irrigated fields regularly – either as workers, or carrying out their domestic chores of providing meals to the workers. In addition, women may also be using the contaminated water to wash clothes. Thus, they are subjected to the same risk factors.

Monitoring the progress of a project against its objectives is about detecting changes, and this information is captured by indicators. The choice of indicators can conceal gender inequality. As argued in the case of the Assuit Burns Centre discussed above, failure to disaggregate statistics such as the number of users of a health centre hides the identity of the service users. Monitoring of service use by gender and age would reveal whether the health needs of non-married women or older women or young men are satisfied.

What impact can be attributed to a particular health project?

How can one prove that a particular change is attributed to a particular project? In some health projects, it is possible to show a linear cause-and-effect relationship. An example would be the reduced incidence of measles among girls and boys, due to an increased vaccination rate. However, as health projects become more complex, so does the process of attribution. It can be difficult to attribute changes in behaviour and attitudes to one project.

Health projects which are planned in a linear way use indicators to measure the project's inputs and outputs, in relation to its stated objectives. However, this narrow, linear approach to monitoring risks attributing all changes to the project and ignoring the impact of wider trends outside the project. In order to avoid the dangers of narrowly focusing on the project alone, various methods of verification are needed. These include monitoring the *context* in which the project takes place, as well as the project itself, and considering the extent to which there is a positive correlation over time between the project's progress, changes in the context, and changes in people's lives. Participatory monitoring, involving men and women in choosing indicators, measuring change, and making correlations, can help to verify correlations.

In addition, such a narrow focus means that any unplanned impact – whether positive or negative – which results from the project is also missed in the monitoring exercise. In the Burns Centre project, the caring attitude of the staff inspired some of the patients' relatives to ask for training in community care for patients and prevention activities. Limiting the monitoring process to looking only at the project objectives would have missed this significant indicator of impact, which shows how the project influenced the wider community and scaled up its effects. Another project, the Abs Centre in Yemen, trains primary health-care workers. Ten years ago, the Abs Centre decided to train a number of women to provide maternity care in an area of high maternal mortality. Through developing the capacity of the women trainees to do this important work, the project challenged the gender norms in the surrounding community. In this project area, women traditionally could not leave the village unaccompanied by a close male relative (father, brother, or husband). Part

of the training was to visit other projects, and to participate in workshops in other towns. The trained women were challenging gender roles in 'professional' health-care provision, traditionally seen as a male domain. Years later, some of the female health workers decided to go without a male escort to the capital city and ask for their salaries at the Ministry of Health. Narrow, linear monitoring would be likely to miss this indicator of women's empowerment. Currently, the health centre is managed by one of these women (Vanni 1993).

What sorts of indicator should be used?

Indicators are used to 'feel the pulse of the project' by measuring changes in various aspects of the project, focusing on process and impact. Choosing the right indicators and the process of making such a choice are important elements of monitoring, in order to stimulate the changes in policy and practice which enhance gender-equitable health gains.

To summarise, indicators may be quantitative, focusing on figures – for example, the number of health units built, the number of girls vaccinated, the number of health-training workshops held, or the numbers of women and men who participated in them. These data are usually collected by keeping regular records and doing formal surveys/questionnaires. In contrast, qualitative indicators present the perceptions of various groups (service providers, policy-makers, donors, and members of the community) on various aspects of the project, as well as changes in the context. Quantitative records will indicate the number of vaccinated girls, while qualitative indicators may refer to service-providers' perception of social change, evidenced by the fact that men are bringing their children for vaccination, and thus taking more responsibility for their children's health. The effects of health training can be measured by the number of trained women and men, as well as by the extent to which the trainer and male participants respect the views of young female participants in the training.

In particular, qualitative indicators can contribute to gender-sensitive monitoring, by focusing on the differing experiences and perceptions of women and men, and challenging the norms of gender relations, both during the course of data collection and in the outcome. These indicators can be collected via informal surveys, participatory methodologies such as semi-structured interviews, focus-group discussions, and other PRA tools. However, it is particularly important not to make the assumption that participatory methods of data collection will auto-matically ensure gender-sensitive data which will reveal gender inequality in a particular context. In fact, some of the PRA tools can be used in a way which excludes women (or some groups of women) from participation. For example, discussions at the time of meal preparation (or other household activities) may exclude women, and women are often uncomfortable to give their views in mixed gatherings (Guijt and Shah 1998).

There is a debate about whether it is valid to use subjective indicators. No research is value-free and objective (Oakley 2000). No indicators are politically neutral, since they are all chosen by an individual or group of people, bringing personal experiences and biases to the research process. Because of this, a single indicator – for example, delay in taking children to a health clinic – will be interpreted differently by different people. The delay may be seen by health professionals as an indicator of mothers' ignorance, while mothers themselves may see it as an indicator of their inability to pay for treatment. If gender-sensitive data have been collected and it is possible to tell how many of the children are girls, a feminist researcher will see a high proportion of

girls among the late attendances as a possible indicator of low prioritisation of health care for girls, suggesting gender inequality. In view of the subjective way in which indicators are chosen and interpreted, it may even be difficult to agree on which indicators point to positive impact, too, since views on changes in the quality of service may differ between men and women, or other social groupings such as young and old. In one village in Uganda, while men and women agreed (in separate focus-group discussions) on many indicators for judging the quality of health services, only women identified the attitude of project staff to HIV-positive people as an important indicator (unpublished Oxfam research in Uganda 1998).

As measures which can be used to stimulate policy and practice changes, indicators should be realistic, operational, and measurable. Chris Roche of Oxfam GB offers an alternative to the idea of SMART indicators, arguing that they should instead be SPICED (Subjective, Participatory, Interpreted, Communicable, Cross-checked and Compared, Empowering, Diverse, and Disaggregated – Roche 1999).

Depending on when the monitoring is taking place, different kinds of indicator may be used:

- **Input indicators** measure the resources in terms of human and financial contribution of the project. For example, how much money has been invested in gender-specific activities, and how much staff time has been dedicated to those activities? How are women involved in the planning and implementing? What training is available for men and women? What medical/health supplies are provided? Is the water pump in a location approved by women? How far is the health centre from the village – could the women walk to it? (Adapted from Beck and Stelcner 1995)

- **Process indicators** measure the delivery of activities and resources, tracking changes towards the stated objectives. These include asking the following questions: who participates in the health project's activities? How are the project activities affected by and how do they affect the seasonal activities of men and women? How many regular meetings are held for health workers? Who participates? Are the meetings held at times when women can participate? How are views of younger and older men and women taken into consideration?

- **Output indicators** measure results which arise during the project and are usually quantifiable. How many health-education sessions have been held? How many men and women participated? How much did the women express their views and how much were they respected? How many girls and boys were vaccinated?

- **Outcome indicators** measure longer-term results of the health project, in terms of improvements in the health of various groups in the community, as well as the extent and nature of their participation, and the implications of all this for changing gender relations and other power relations in the community. What are the improvements in health of men, women, girls, and boys? Who was not affected, and why? What has changed in the decision-making processes in households and wider community institutions, in terms of women's involvement in the process?

Conclusion

Monitoring of health interventions can focus on organisational performance, the impact of health policy, and the process and impact of health projects and programmes. Monitoring should start at the same time as a particular policy, project, programme, or organisational process begins. It starts with identifying clear objectives and baseline information. Then the following steps should be taken:

1. Identification of indicators through agreement between various stakeholders, especially planners and implementers, on a small set of basic indicators. These indicators should be designed to reveal differences between women's and men's roles, and inequalities in gender relations, which may lead to different outcomes for women and men. It may be possible to involve women and men from the community in defining the indicators, and what they signify. However, there should be flexibility to allow this set to be adapted and verified, and to include other indicators, as work progresses.

2. Data collection of quantitative and qualitative information and indicators, via formal survey, records, and participatory methodologies.

3. Analysis of the collected data, to verify indicators and interpret the data, and make recommendations. Gender analysis of the data is crucial, to identify gaps and achievements in terms of gender equity. Involving women and men from the community in interpreting and analysing the data can be a useful verifying tool.

4. Presenting the data in a useful way and sharing the documents with other stakeholders.

5. Use of the monitoring data to stimulate policy and practice changes necessary to achieve the main objectives.

Governments, NGOs, and international development agencies, including those working in the health sector, do not usually invest sufficient resources in monitoring and evaluation. All organisations involved in health interventions need to recognise that monitoring and evaluation are valuable tools to stimulate policy and practice changes which will promote good health for women as well as men. In conclusion, a successful gender-sensitive system of monitoring and evaluation needs adequate human and financial resources in order to function, and a commitment to building the capacity of health professionals and other staff in terms of gender-sensitive planning, implementation, and monitoring and evaluation. It is crucial for organisations to recognise that systematic monitoring and evaluation, and particularly approaches that involve women and men from the community in participatory methodologies, are demanding in terms of time. Sufficient resources should be dedicated to developing these systems.

Dr Mohga Smith is Health Adviser in Oxfam GB's Policy Department, Oxfam GB, 174 Banbury Road, Oxford OX2 7DZ, UK. E-mail: msmith@oxfam.org.uk

Notes

1 Doyal, draft framework for designing national health policies with an integrated gender perspective, http://www.un.org/womenwatch/daw/csw/papers1.htm

References

Beck, T. and Stelcner, M. (1995) *Guide To Gender Sensitive Indicators*, CIDA.

Gilson, L. (1997) 'Review paper: the lessons of user-fee experience in Africa', *Health Policy and Planning* 12.

Guijt, I. and M. Kaul Shah (eds) (1998) *The Myth Of Community: Gender Issues In Participatory Development*, London: IT Publications.

Hartmann, B. (1987) *Reproductive Rights and Wrongs. The Global Politics of Population Control and Contraceptive Choice*, New York: Harper and Row

March, C., Smyth, I., and M. Mukhopadhay (1999) *A Guide To Gender Analysis Frameworks*, Oxford: Oxfam Publications.

Moser, C. (no date) 'The Impact of Recession and Structural Adjustment at the Micro-level: Low-income Women and their Households in Guayaquil, Ecuador', New York: UNICEF.

Oakley, A. (2000) *Experiments in Knowing: Gender and Method in the Social Sciences*, Cambridge: Polity Press.

Roche, C. (1999) *Impact Assessment For Development Agencies: Learning to Value Change*, Oxford: Oxfam Publications.

Smith, M. K. (1997) 'A Tool or a Toll: The Effectiveness of Growth Monitoring on the Nutritional Status of Children Under Five in Poor Urban Communities in the Developing World', unpublished dissertation, University of Bristol, UK.

Standing, H. (1997) 'Gender and equity in health sector reform programmes: a review', *Health Policy and Planning* 12: 1-18.

Standing, H. (2000) 'Gender Impacts of Health Reforms – The Current State Of Policy and Implementation', unpublished paper for ALAMES meeting, Havana, Cuba 3-7 July.

Vanni, V.F.K. (1993) 'Combating inequality', *Health Action*, 2: 10.

Resources

Compiled by Erin Murphy Graham

Publications

Sex, Gender and Health (1999), Tessa M. Pollard and Susan Brin Hyatt (eds), Cambridge University Press, Cambridge CB2 2RU, UK. This collection brings together the work of biological and social anthropologists to explain the different experiences of sickness and health of women and men in societies all over the world. Argues that an understanding of science and culture, using notions of biological 'sex' and socially constructed 'gender', is essential for furthering this analysis.

Women's Health: From Womb to Tomb (1991), Penny Kane, Macmillan, Houndmills, Basingstoke, Hampshire RG21 6XS, UK. This book moves beyond a focus on reproductive health alone, to examine the many differences between men's and women's health at all stages of life. Chapters focus on trends in women's health, explanations for women's health advantage, women and illness, social and economic health differences, female health in childhood and early adulthood, and health in the middle and later years.

The Health of Women: A Global Perspective (1993), Marge Koblinsky, Judith Timyan, and Jill Gay, Westview Press, 12 Hid's Copse Road, Cumnor Hill, Oxford OX2 9JJ, UK. The product of the 1991 National Council for International Health Conference on 'Women's Health: The Action Agenda', the book discusses the information and services women need to improve their health and the context in which they live their lives. Twelve chapters focus on specific issues including abortion, women's mental health, family planning and reproductive health, women's nutrition, and the importance of listening to women when they discuss their health needs.

Gender and the Social Construction of Illness (1997), Judith Lorber, Sage Publications, 6 Bonhill Street, London EC2A 4PU, UK. Explores the interaction between gender as a social institution on one hand, and western medicine as a social institution on the other. Focusing on illnesses that are considered in western medicine to be purely physical, Lorber brings a feminist viewpoint to analyse issues of power and politics. Discusses gender and HIV/AIDS, premenstrual syndrome, and menopause, and concludes with a chapter on feminist health care.

The Health Gap, Beyond Pregnancy and Reproduction (1996), Jennifer Kitts and Janet Hatcher Roberts, International Development Research Center (IDRC), PO Box 8500, Ottawa, ON, Canada K1G 3H9.

When health research has addressed the concerns of women, it has tended to focus on their reproductive health needs. This book redresses the balance by adopting a holistic approach to women's health. It identifies and addresses key gaps in research: women and AIDS, tropical disease, the working environment, and barriers to health care. It also identifies new and emerging themes in women's health, and sets the priorities for future action.

Where Women Have No Doctor (1997), The Hesperian Foundation, 1919 Addison Street, Suite 304, Berkeley, California 94704, USA.

This guide for use by women at community level combines self-help medical information with an understanding of the ways poverty, discrimination, and cultural beliefs limit women's health and access to care. Developed with community groups and medical experts from more than 30 countries, it uses simple language and pictures. It is useful for anyone interested in improving women's health through understanding, treating, and preventing their health problems.

Women in Pain: Gender and Morbidity in Mexico (1994), Kaja Finkler, University of Pennsylvania Press, 4200 Pine Street, Philadelphia, PA 19104-4011, USA.

During studies spanning 20 years, the author lived with various Mexican families, participated in their daily activities and was trained as a spiritual healer – all of which gave her the opportunity to observe women's daily lives and social interactions. This book is about how the Mexican women's lives she observed are intertwined with their experience of sickness and health. It begins with chapters on women's health and the context of the study, and then includes ten portraits of Mexican women who discuss their experiences of sickness and health.

Taking Sides: Clashing Views on Controversial Issues in Gender Studies (1998), Alison D. Spalding (ed.), Dushkin/McGraw Hill, Guildford, CT 06437, USA.

A debate-style reader designed to introduce controversial issues in gender studies. The fourth part focuses on gender and health, with chapters on: 'Is there a male sex bias in medicine?' 'Is premenstrual syndrome a clear medical condition?' 'Do women suffer from post-abortion syndrome?' and 'Should ritual female genital surgery be regulated worldwide?'

Gender and Mental Health (1999), Pauline Prior, Macmillan.

This book offers a gendered and cross-cultural analysis of the experience of mental distress and of society's response to it. The book explores the relationship between socially accepted views of normality and psychiatric diagnosis for men and women. Draws on the latest debates in masculinity theory, as well as feminist and sociological explanations, to discuss the over-representation of women in measures of mental illness.

Gender and Health: An International Perspective (1996), Carolyn F. Sargent and Caroline B. Brettell, Prentice Hall, Upper Saddle River, NJ 07458, USA.

A comprehensive guide to gender and health issues from an international perspective. Part V focuses on 'Gender, healing and the social production of women'. Includes a chapter on refugee women from El Salvador describing their experiences of trauma and political violence, and the health consequences of this trauma.

'Some Men Really Are Useless': The Role of Participating in a Women's Project, Empowerment and Gender in the Context of Two Zimbabwean Women's Organizations (1997), Geeske Hoogenboezem, Third World Center/ Development Studies, Catholic University, PO Box 9104 NL 6500 HE, Nijmegen, The Netherlands.

Profiles the Health Information Project in Zimbabwe and the interplay between women's participation and their empowerment. Argues that the workings of gender, the subtle mechanisms and manipulations of power and intersections between social, cultural, symbolic, and economic spheres of life should be allowed for in an appropriate description of the empowerment approach.

Monitoring Family Planning & Reproductive Rights: A Manual for Empowerment (1997), Anita Hardon, Ann Mutua, Sandra Kabir, and Elly Engelkes, Zed Books, 7 Cynthia Street, London N1 9JF, UK.

Provides a framework for researching family planning provision in different cultural settings and offers NGOs and other health research bodies how to design such projects and provides indicators for quality assessment. Chapters explore the full range of skills required to conduct research, from choosing the size of the sample to processing the final data.

Health Communication: Lessons from Family Planning and Reproductive Health (1997), Phyllis Tilson Piotrow, D. Lawrence Kincaid, Jose G. Rimon II, and Ward Rinehart, Praeger Publishers, 88 Post Road West, Westport, CT 06881, USA.

Argues that with the growth of mass media and the scientific methods to measure its impact, communication now plays a crucial role in social change, especially in Latin America, Africa, and Asia. This book centres on the lessons learned about effective family planning communication over the past 15 years and offers several examples of how to plan for and evaluate effective family planning communication internationally.

Making a Difference: Women's Reproductive Health, Rights, Empowerment and Male Involvement (1998), Association for Reproductive and Family Health, 13 Ajayi Osungbekun Street, Ikolaba GRA, PO Box 30259, Ibadan, Nigeria.

Presents the achievements, key evaluation findings, and lessons learned in project implementation of the Women's Reproductive Health, Rights, Empowerment, and Male Involvement project. Could inform similar projects in other settings.

Evaluating Health Promotion: Practice and Methods (2000), Margaret Thorogood and Yolande Coombes, Oxford University Press, Great Clarendon Street, Oxford OX2 6DP, UK.

This book discusses the concepts of health promotion and evaluation in their historical context. It highlights key issues in the evaluation of health promotion interventions, several qualitative and quantitative methods that are commonly used, and experiences in the implementation of health evaluation in a variety of settings.

Improving Family Planning Evaluation: A Step-by-Step Guide for Managers and Evaluators (1992), José García-Núñez, Kumarian Press, 630 Oakwood Avenue, Suite 119, West Hartford, CT 06110-1529, USA.

This guidebook attempts to simplify the daunting task of designing and implementing program evaluations, particularly in family planning programs. Describes the evaluation methodologies that will satisfy the reporting needs of donors and constituents and the ways in which evaluations are used in cost-effective project planning. A helpful resource for practitioners and evaluation specialists.

Reproductive Health in Developing Countries: Expanding Dimensions, Building Solutions (1997), Amy O. Tsui, Judith N. Wasserheit, and John G. Haaga (eds), National Academy Press, 2101 Constitution Ave NW, Washington, DC 20418, USA.

Focuses on sexually-transmitted diseases, unintended pregnancies, infertility, and other reproductive problems in developing countries. Discusses what is known about the effectiveness of interventions in four areas: infection-free sex, intended pregnancies and births, healthy pregnancy and delivery, and healthy sexuality (including sexual violence and female genital mutilation).

Voluntary Action in Health and Population: The Dynamic of Social Transition (2000), Sunil Misra (ed.), Sage Publications.

This book brings together 14 case studies of action research projects undertaken by voluntary organisations in the field of health and family planning. They cover projects in different socio-cultural situations across ten different states in India. Attempts to assist in the formulation of methodologies and long-term strategies to transform positive change into enduring social behaviour.

Women's Reproductive Rights in Developing Countries (1999), Vijayan K. Pillai and Guang-Zhen Wang, Ashgate Publishing Ltd., Gower House, Croft Road, Aldershot, Hants GU11 3HR, UK.

Presents an empirical model of reproductive rights in developing countries, encompassing three explanations of reproductive rights: that reproductive rights are negatively related to population growth; that gender equality has a positive effect on reproductive rights; and that women's education has a positive effect on reproductive rights. The authors argue that value-based structural changes play an important role in improving reproductive rights.

Private Decisions, Public Debate: Women, Reproduction and Population (1994), Panos Institute, 9 White Lion Street, London N1 9PD, UK.

In this book, 15 journalists from Africa, Asia, and Latin America present the views of women and report on subjects such as son preference, female genital mutilation, unauthorized sterilisations, untreated STDs, HIV infection, and the influence of Catholicism and Islam, all of which affect reproductive decision making.

Population and Reproductive Rights: Feminist Perspectives from the South (1994), Sonia Correa, Zed Books.

Brings a critical feminist perspective to the conventional debates around population issues. Examines the interlinking of economic processes, demographic dynamics and women's lives, as well as the detrimental effects on women of past and present fertility management policies. Correa argues for the indivisibility of health and rights, and identifies the challenges which women in the South need to tackle. Lastly, she suggests appropriate strategies for political action by the international women's movement around these issues.

Power, Reproduction and Gender: The Intergenerational Transfer of Knowledge (1997), Wendy Harcourt (ed.), Zed Books.

Explores the issues of health, empowerment, sexuality, and reproductive rights – issues, it argues, that are central to the on-going international development debate on population and gender. It asks whether we can and should change cultural knowledge, codes, and practice related to reproductive behaviour, sexuality, and gender relations. Chapters focus on these issues in Africa, Latin America, and Asia.

Unwanted Pregnancies and Public Policy: An International Perspective (1994), Hector Correa (ed.), Nova Science Publishers, Inc., 6080 Jericho Turnpike, Suite 207, Commack, NY 11725, USA.

A comprehensive volume that includes papers analysing the problems associated with unwanted pregnancies and their outcomes from an international perspective. Individual chapters focus on adolescent fertility in Africa, illegal induced abortion in Brazil, female infanticide in India, the consequences of unwanted pregnancies in Bolivia, and an international comparison of abortion laws and practice.

Reproductive Health in Refugee Situations: An Inter-Agency Field Manual (1999), Women, Ink, 777 United Nations Plaza, New York, NY 10017, USA.

This inter-agency field manual on reproductive health in refugee situations is the result of a collaborative effort of many UN agencies, governmental and non-governmental organisations, and refugees themselves. This manual is based on the normative, technical guidance of the World Health Organization and addresses topics such as family planning, STDs, safe motherhood, and sexual and gender-based violence. Also available online at http://www.ippf.org/resource/refugeehealth/manual/index.htm

Pregnancy Outcome Among Displaced and Non-Displaced Women in Bosnia and Herzegovina (1996), International Centre for Migration and Health, 11 Route du Nant d'Avril, CH-1214 Geneva, Switzerland.

A report based on the findings of an international group of experts convened by ICMH in October 1995 to assess how the war in Bosnia and Herzegovina and the associated displacement of women affected pregnancy outcomes. Documents the pregnancy experience of displaced and local women in Sarajevo, and proposes steps that could be taken to improve reproductive health in general, and especially health during pregnancy, in similar situations elsewhere.

Refugee Women (1995) in Refugees (100(II)) a journal published by the United Nations High Commission for Refugees, CP 2500, 1211 Geneva 2, Switzerland.

This edition of the journal *Refugees*, a quarterly magazine that describes refugee events and issues, focuses on women refugees, including their health needs. One article describes an ambitious reproductive health program for Rwandan refugees in Tanzania that targets everything from safer childbirth to the prevention of sexually transmitted diseases.

Reproductive Health Matters, Blackwell Science LTD, Journal Subscriptions, PO Box 88, Oxford OX2 0NE, UK.

Reproductive Health Matters is an international, peer-reviewed journal, published twice a year. It offers in-depth analysis of reproductive health matters from a women-centred perspective. Articles are written by and for women's health advocates, researchers, service providers, policy-makers, and those in related fields with an interest in women's health. Its aim is to promote laws, policies, research, and services that meet women's reproductive health needs and support women's right to decide whether, when and how to have children. Each issue focuses on a main theme, and also contains topical papers on other aspects of sexual and reproductive health.

Preventing and Mitigating AIDS in Sub-Saharan Africa: Research and Data Priorities for the Social and Behavioral Sciences (1996), National Research Council, National Academy Press, 2101 Constitution Ave. NW, Washington DC 20418, USA.

Details the current state of the AIDS epidemic in Africa and what is known about the behaviours that contribute to the transmission of the HIV virus. It discusses what research is needed and what is possible to design more effective prevention programs, working with both men and women.

Gender Relations and AIDS: Women and Youths' Capacity to Fight Against HIV/AIDS in Tegeta Village of Dar es Salaam Region, Preliminary Findings, Feddy Mwanga, Society for Women and Aids in Africa, PO Box 65081, Dar es Salaam, Tanzania.

This study presents the findings from a qualitative investigation in Dar es Salaam on what women and youth are doing to prevent the spread of HIV / AIDS. Issues such as lack of women's control over sex with their partners, stigmas around condom use, and gender roles and cultural values are discussed. While this study is specific to Dar es Salaam, it serves as an example to other researchers and practitioners interested in investigating how women are resisting HIV / AIDS.

Adolescents in Death-Defying Sex-Search: Integrating the Role of Constructions of Masculinity in a HIV/AIDS/STD Education Programme Designed for an Urban Tanzanian Context. A Gender Assessment Study (1997), Ludo Bok, Third World Center / Development Studies, Catholic University, PO Box 9104, NL 6500 HE, Nijmegen, The Netherlands.

Explores the way future HIV / AIDS / STD education programmes could deal with the behaviour of adolescent boys and the ways masculinity is constructed in order to change unsafe sexual behaviour of adolescents. Concludes that future education programmes must target not only adolescents, but parents, religious leaders, health workers, and governmental institutions.

What Makes Women Sick: Gender and the Political Economy of Health (1995), Lesley Doyal, Macmillan.

Rather than focusing on the biology of women's bodies, this book demonstrates the limitations of such an approach and explores the economic, social, and cultural influences in women's lives that can make them sick. Section II focuses on the 'hazards of hearth and home' and includes chapters on cross-cultural perspectives on domestic work, the occupational hazards of unpaid labour, and women's labour in the household economy.

Gender Research on Urbanisation, Planning, Housing and Everyday Life (1995), Sylvia Sithole-Fundire, Agnes Zhou, Anita Larsson, and Ann Schlyter (eds), Zimbabwe Women's Resource Centre and Network, 288c Herbert Chitepo Avenue, PO Box 2192, Harare, Zimbabwe.

Presents papers based on the research carried out during the first phase of a research programme by the same title, which aims to support gender research within the areas of urbanisation, planning, housing, and everyday life.

The Poor Die Young: Housing and Health in Third World Cities (1990), Jorge E. Hardoy, Sandy Cairncross, and David Satterthwaite (eds), Earthscan, 3 Endsleigh Street, London WC1H 0DD, UK.

Attempts to promote a greater understanding and increased awareness about the effects of the home environment on health and wellbeing. Argues that these issues are intertwined with social factors such as poverty, educational achievement, the role of women, the right to property, nutrition, migration, and democratic governance. Individual chapters focus on the role of women in an experimental waste collection project in N'Djamena, Chad, and housing and health in three squatter settlements in India.

Gender, Health, and Sustainable Development (1993), Pandu Wijeryaratne, Lori Jones Arsenault, Janet Hatcher Roberts, and Jennifer Kitts (eds), International Development Research Center (IDRC).

The first section of these conference proceedings focuses on AIDS, sexually transmitted diseases, and gender. The second discusses tropical diseases (such as malaria) and gender. The third focuses on environmental stress, production activities, health, and gender – including a chapter on environmental degradation, gender, and health in Ghana. Finally, social issues, gender, and health are discussed.

Organisations

International Centre for Migration and Health, 11 Route du Nant d'Avril, CH - 1214 Geneva, Switzerland. Tel: + (41 22) 783 10 80; fax: + (41 22) 783 10 87;
E-mail: ICMH@worldcom.ch
http://www.icmh.ch/
ICMH was established in 1995, as part of a joint initiative by IOM, the University of Geneva, and WHO, in response to the need for more research, policy, and training in the area of migration and health. ICMH has been designated as a WHO Collaborating Centre for Health-Related Issues Among People Displaced by Disasters. Its particular areas of interest include the impact of migration on household structure and family life and its effect on the health of vulnerable groups such as women, children, and the elderly; and the impact of migration on the spread of infectious diseases.

The International Women's Health Coalition, 24 East 21 Street New York, NY 10010.
http://www.iwhc.org
IWHC believes that global wellbeing, and social and economic justice, can only be achieved by ensuring women's human rights, health, and equality. Through a variety of programs and activities, IWHC seeks to ensure that women are equally and effectively engaged in decisions that concern their sexual and reproductive rights and health; that women experience a healthy and satisfying sexual life free from discrimination, coercion, and violence; that women can make free and informed choices about childbearing; and that women have access to the information and services they need to enhance and protect their health.

The Program on Women, Health and Development at the Pan American Health Organisation, Division of Health and Human Development, Pan American Health Organization, 525 23rd Street NW, Washington, DC 20037, USA.
Tel: + (202) 974 3405; fax: + (202) 974 3671;
E-mail: hdw@paho.org
The mandate of PAHO's Women, Health and Development Program (HDW) is to provide technical co-operation to member countries to promote equitable and sustainable development with a gender perspective. HDW seeks identify and reduce inequalities between women and men that are unnecessary, unjust, and avoidable with regard to: health outcomes and their determinants; access to resources and quality care that serve the specific needs of women and men from different social groups; allocation of public and private health resources. In Spanish and English.

International Planned Parenthood Federation, Regent's College, Inner Circle, Regent's Park, London NW1 4NS, UK.
Tel: + 44 (0)20 7487 7900; fax: + 44 (0)20 7487 7950
E-mail: info@ippf.org
http://www.ippf.org/
The International Planned Parenthood Federation (IPPF) links national autonomous Family Planning Associations in over 150 countries worldwide. IPPF and its member associations are committed to promoting the right of women and men to decide freely the number and spacing of their children and the right to the highest possible level of sexual

and reproductive health.

InterAction, 1717 Massachusetts Ave. NW, Suite 701, Washington, DC 20036, USA.
Tel: + (202) 667 8227; fax: + (202) 667-5362
E-mail: ia@interaction.org
A coalition of more than 150 non-profit organisations, concerned with international relief and development, working worldwide. Distributes information on development, refugees, advocacy, and disaster response. InterAction member organisations promote economic develop-ment and self-reliance, improve health and education, provide relief to victims of disasters and wars, assist refugees, advance human rights, protect the environment, address population concerns, advocate for more just public policies and increase understanding and co-operation between people. Women are central to many of these programmes, and special efforts are made to promote women's participation and equity.

The Population Council, 1 Dag Hammarskjöld Plaza, New York, NY 10017-2201, USA
Tel: + (212) 339 0500
E-mail: Pubinfo@popcouncil.org
The Population Council is a non-profit research NGO, established in 1952. The Council analyses population issues and trends, conducts biomedical research to develop new contraceptives, works with public and private agencies to improve the quality and outreach of family planning and reproductive health services, helps governments to influence demographic behaviour, communicates the results of research in the population field to appropriate audiences, and helps build research capacities in developing countries.

The World Health Organisation, Avenue Appia 20, 1211 Geneva 27, Switzerland.
Tel: + (41 22) 791 21 11;
fax: + (41 22) 791 31 11
http://www.who.int/home-page/
The main objective of the World Health Organization is the attainment by all peoples of the highest possible level of health. Health, as defined by the WHO constitution, is a state of complete physical, mental, and social wellbeing and not merely the absence of disease or infirmity. The site gives insight into WHO programs and activities.

Electronic Resources

The Women's Health Department Home Page of the WHO
http://www.who.int/frh-whd/index.html
The official website of the WHO women's health division. Contains information on women and HIV/AIDS, FGM, reproductive health, and violence against women. Also contains links to other sites and organi-sations dealing with women's health issues and WHO publications on women's health including technical reports and working papers.

WHO Women's Health Fact Sheets
http://www.who.int/frh-whd/FactSheets/English/index.htm
Available in French and English, this site has fact sheets on topics including FGM, women and HIV/AIDS, emergency contra-ception, breast cancer, women and microbicides, pregnancy, and women and mental health.

Secure and Promote Women's Health (an online forum sponsored by WomenWatch Beijing +5 Global Forum, 6 September -- 15 October 1999)
http://www.un.org/womenwatch/forums/beijing5/health/health.htm
This online forum addressed the following questions: Has there been progress in promoting women's health? What are the obstacles? What must be done in the future? Reports from the various working groups and on-line discussions are available at this site. Available in French, Spanish, and English.

Online Dialogue on Women and Health, Follow-up to the Beijing Conference on Women
http://www.un.org/womenwatch/daw/csw/wohealth.htm
The United Nations Division for the Advancement of Women conducted a three-week on-line conference/dialogue on women and health, proceedings of which are detailed on this site. Participants discussed good practices as well as identified obstacles to implementing the Beijing Platform for Action. Discussion papers, the expert group meeting, and discussions are included.

The Global Reproductive Health Forum @ Harvard (GRHF)
http://www.hsph.harvard.edu/Organizations/healthnet/
An internet networking project that aims to encourage the proliferation of critical, democratic discussions about reproductive health and gender on the net. The project provides interactive electronic forums, located in Southern countries, which hope to encourage the participation of under served groups, and distributes reproductive health and rights materials from a variety of perspectives through the website.

The Reproductive Health Outlook (RHO)
http://www.rho.org/
Provides summaries of up-to-date information, links to the best in-depth reproductive health information on the web, and the chance to communicate with international experts and peers through Community Forum message boards. RHO is especially designed for reproductive health program managers and decision makers working in low-resource settings.

Videos

The Road to Change (2000), VHS, 45 minutes, English and French editions.
World Health Organization, Distribution and Sales, CH-1211 Geneva 27, Switzerland.
Tel: + (41 22) 791 24 76
E-mail: bookorders@who.ch
From the huts of Africa to the cities of Manchester and San Francisco, this film makes a compelling case for the need to end FGM. It also places FGM within the context of other practices, throughout history and in different civilizations, that have attempted to control the status and sexuality of women. As the film repeatedly stresses, the practice cannot be effectively addressed until its traditional and cultural significance is fully understood.

Generation 2000: Changing Girls' Realities, VHS, 15 minutes.
International Women's Health Coalition, 24 East 21st Street, New York, NY 10010, USA.
Tel: + (212) 979 8500; fax: + (212) 979 9009
A film about adolescent girls in Nigeria, conceived and narrated by Jane Fonda in collaboration with the International Women's Health Coalition (IWHC). Portrays three organizations working with girls in Nigeria: Girls' Power Initiative in Calabar, Action Health, Incorporated in Lagos, and the Adolescent Health and Information Project in Kano. Illustrates how programs focusing on adolescents' reproductive health and rights are effective

and accepted by parents, schools, religious leaders, and government officials in Nigeria.

Lifelines (online video clips)
http://www.ippf.org/videos/index.htm
Lifelines is a series of 12 sixty-second clips shot on 35mm for television broadcast and cinema exhibition. Based on International Planned Parenthood Federation's Charter on Sexual and Reproductive Rights, the storylines illustrate what the denial of reproductive rights means in reality for women around the world.

The Women's Agenda: Kenya/UGANDA, ZebraLink Communications Limited, PO Box 34696, Nairobi, Kenya.
E-mail: dommleyo@tchuinet.com
This video documentary adopts a continental African perspective with examples drawn from Kenya and Uganda on the progress women have made in implementing the agenda set out in Beijing in 1995. Includes a discussion of health, girls, and women's empowerment. It concludes by highlighting women's agendas for the future.

Courses

Gender Health and Communicable Disease, Liverpool School of Tropical Medicine, Pembroke Place, Liverpool L3 5QA, UK.
Contact Phil Hinds; tel: + 44 (0) 151 708 9393; fax: + 44 (0) 151 708 8733;
E-mail: hinds@liv.ac.uk
http://www.liv.ac.uk/lstm/lstm.html
This annual short course aims to enhance the capacity of policy-makers to analyse and address gender inequalities in health and health care in developing countries. The course has a specific focus on gender in infectious diseases such as TB, malaria, and sexually transmitted infections, and their implications for health systems development.
International Summer School, Refugee Studies Centre (RSC), Refugee Studies

Centre, Queen Elizabeth House, University of Oxford, 21 St Giles, Oxford, OX1 3LA, UK.
Tel: + 44 (0) 1865 270722;
fax: + 44 (0) 1865 270721;
E-mail: RSC@qeh.ox.ac.uk
The RSC's annual International Summer School is a three-week-long course that provides a broad perspective on the issues of forced migration and humanitarian assistance. It combines lecturing and active learning methods, which allow experienced practitioners to study, learn, reflect, and share their experience with others in a setting removed from the day-to-day pressures of work.

IPPF/GTZ Course on Population and Development, The Global Advocacy Division, International Planned Parenthood Federation.
Tel: + 44 (0) 207 487 7864/7856;
fax: + 44 (0) 207 487 7865;
E-mail: cambridge@ippf.org
http://www.ippf.org/resource/courses/camb2000/index.htm
An intensive two-week residential course held annually in Cambridge in July for professionals in the field of family planning and sexual and reproductive health.